AIDS:
Living and Dying
with Hope

Issues in Pastoral Care

Walter J. Smith, S.J.

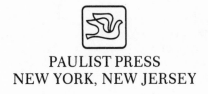

PAULIST PRESS
NEW YORK, NEW JERSEY

For R.G.H., Jr. and the nameless other persons with AIDS whose courage, faith, and love continually strengthen those who are privileged to care for them.

For Joseph D. Devlin, S.J., Rector of the Jesuit Community at Fairfield University, whose sensitivity, encouragement, and un-failing support have exemplified what pastoral care can be.

Excerpts from *The Screaming Room,* copyright © 1986 by Barbara Peabody are used by permission of Oak Tree Publications, Inc. of San Diego, CA. Passages from *Good-bye, I Love You,* copyright © 1986 by Carol Lynn Pearson are cited with the permission of Random House, Inc. Quotations from *When Someone You Love Has AIDS,* copyright © 1986 by BettyClare Moffat are used with the permission of NAL Penguin Inc. Citations from *AIDS: The Spiritual Dilemma,* copyright © 1987 by John E. Fortunato are reproduced with the permission of Harper & Row, Publishers, Inc.

Library of Congress Cataloging-in-Publication Data

Smith, Walter J.
   AIDS : living and dying with hope.

      1. AIDS (Disease)—Patients—Pastoral counseling of.
I. Title.
BV4460.7.S65 1988   259'.4
ISBN 0-8091-3000-9 (pbk.)

Published by Paulist Press
997 Macarthur Boulevard
Mahwah, New Jersey 07430

Printed and bound in the United States of America

Contents

Preface

The contemporary story began silently in the early to mid-1970s when the global spread of a virus appears to have started. In the summer of 1981 the Center for Disease Control (CDC) cited in its weekly newsletter five cases of an unusual pneumonia in young homosexual men in Los Angeles. Some of these patients also had a cancer rarely seen in younger persons. By the early months of 1982 the CDC was referring to cases with these symptoms as Acquired Immunodeficiency Syndrome, which quickly was understood by its acronym, AIDS.

Since that time the AIDS story has become a part of our common experience. In the intervening years, the international press and electronic media have chronicled the spread of a disease which has become a pandemic. Despite the medical sophistication which characterizes our technologically advanced societies in these final decades of the twentieth century, AIDS presents us with frightening challenges. Although there are promising technical and scientific advances, at this time there is no cure for AIDS and no vaccine to prevent AIDS. AIDS has mobilized the international scientific community not only to seek a cure for the disease, but also to prevent and control its spread.

The worldwide medical community was slow to recognize the broad spectrum of ways in which AIDS would affect individuals, families, and societies. Now in the latter years of the 1980s we are beginning to assess accurately the costs in terms of human suffering, health care, and social impact. People who have been exposed to the virus are uncertain about their future health. Others worry about becoming infected. Family life is disrupted when children, mothers, or fathers develop either the clinical illness called AIDS or some related symptoms associated with the virus. When a significant number of productive 20–40 year old women and men in industrialized and developing countries throughout the world become ill, require extensive medical interventions, and eventually die, the social and economic fabric is stretched.

AIDS is not simply a medical problem of increasing magnitude; it is also a spiritual and psychosocial concern. The international health community was slow in identifying and responding to the AIDS pandemic. Women and men from different faith traditions have likewise been slow in mobilizing their resources and skills to address this new pastoral concern.

Persons facing a life-threatening illness like AIDS or ARC (AIDS-Related Complex) often seek support from individuals providing pastoral care. This is true both for persons who have had previous affiliations with churches and synagogues, and for those who have been estranged from traditional religious practice. Life-threatening illnesses engage a variety of cognitive, emotional, and spiritual processes. Pastoral care of persons with AIDS (PWAs) or persons with ARC (PWARCs) requires a particular understanding and sensitivity to these various levels of need.

A diagnosis of AIDS or ARC causes many people to experience acute crisis. Human crises are not always pathological; for many people crises are opportunities for change, action, and growth. Crises stimulate individuals to ask new questions about the meaning of their lives and to seek new intellectual and behavioral responses. In his celebrated book, *The Concept of Dread* (1944), Søren Kierkegaard describes crises as leading to "the moment when a person suddenly grasps the meaning of some important event in the past or future in the present, this grasping of the new meaning always presents the possibility and necessity of some personal decision, some shift in gestalt, some new orientation of the person toward the world and the future."

In the face of crises, individuals not uncommonly seek pastoral assistance and are receptive to support, understanding, and guidance. During a crisis, a person usually has a heightened desire to be helped and may be more susceptible to influence than during periods of relatively stable functioning. The pastor is strategically positioned to be a significant resource to an individual in crisis.

Pastors come into contact with persons at these highly critical and sensitive moments. When the precipitating crisis is a diagnosis related to AIDS, there is much that a skilled pastor can do to assist the person not only to regain emotional equilibrium, but to use the crisis event as a way to restructure effectively his or her life. How is a pastor to understand his or her role in responding to an individual in crisis?

In his classic study, *Principles of Preventive Psychiatry*, Gerald Caplan (1964) defined crisis as a condition "provoked when a person faces an obstacle to important life goals that is, for a time, insurmountable through the utilization of customary methods of problem solving." According to this model, a person will first attempt to handle the "obstacle" by resorting to customary problem-solving strategies. When these prove ineffective, he or she will be open to other resources, among which are pastoral counseling and other forms of pastoral care. The sensitivity and skill of these pastoral interventions can affect significantly the course of personal adjustment.

Another way of understanding the precipitating event that brings a person in crisis to seek pastoral assistance can be explained by cognitive theory. Crisis is understood as a breakdown in thinking and reasoning that occurs because of physical and psychological overload. The diagnosis of AIDS or ARC sets the mind racing. Emotionally taxing information, coupled with physical stresses associated with the illness, interrupts coping and problem-solving abilities. A person seeks help to sort out much of the dissonant thoughts and associated feelings. A pastor is often the person to whom an individual turns for guidance and support. The pastor's principal function is to respond to the person's need for understanding and to help him or her process the information so that he or she will be able to continue to maintain control over the course of the illness.

Crises tend to be temporary and self-limiting experiences. Likewise, intervention efforts are frequently of brief duration.

However, in the case of a crisis precipitated by a life-threatening disease like AIDS, the crisis is extended. Once a pastor responds effectively to a PWA, it can be anticipated that the relationship could become intensive and longterm.

In this book we shall consider some of the issues involved in the pastoral care of PWAs and PWARCs. Pastoral care is the most broadly defined activity of those involved in religious ministry. It encompasses not only sacramental and liturgical ministrations, but also techniques of crisis management, spiritual direction, pastoral counseling, psychotherapy, and related practices. While pastors are appropriately educated and skilled to assume some of these functions, the AIDS pandemic presents challenges for which some pastors feel unprepared.

For almost twenty years I have been involved as a clinician in the care of dying persons and their families. Since 1982, that practice has included an increasing number of persons with AIDS. Many of the cases included in this book are from my clinical and pastoral experiences. The rest have been excerpted from published works or from the experiences of other pastors who care for persons with AIDS. Details of these cases have been altered to preserve the privacy of the individuals and families involved, as well as the identity of the clergy who have ministered to them. These combined stories provide a springboard for considering strategies for intervention with persons in similar circumstances. They vividly remind us that caring for persons with AIDS, in their living and in their dying, is a profoundly human and spiritual engagement.

My own professional work and ministry has been supported by the people I have been fortunate to assist. Whatever insight and direction this book can provide for others engaged in the ministry of compassionate service is directly attributable to those whose stories are told herein. Persons with AIDS have much to teach us about living and dying.

I am grateful to the staff at Paulist Press for their interest in the persons whose stories tell us what pastoral care entails. Donald F. Brophy, Managing Editor, expressed enthusiasm for this project from its inception, and his commitment to this book has been consistent. I wish to thank Joseph Devlin, S.J., Thomas

McGrath, S.J., and Walter Woods for their careful reading of the manuscript and for their helpful suggestions. My gratitude is most humbly expressed to those whose struggles to live and die with AIDS have made this book a necessity.

> *Blessed be the Lord!*
> *for God has heard the voice of my pleading.*
> *The Lord is my strength and my shield;*
> *in God my heart trusts;*
> *so I am helped, and my heart exults,*
> *and with my song I give thanks to God.*
>
> *The Lord is the strength of God's people,*
> *The Lord is the saving refuge of God's anointed.*
> *Oh save your people, and bless your heritage;*
> *be their shepherd and carry them forever.*
>
> *Psalm 28:6–9*

1

Acquired Immunodeficiency Syndrome: The Disease

Effective pastoral care of any individual with a life-threatening illness requires that the pastor have a basic, yet competent understanding of the disease afflicting the person, its course, and its treatment. In attempting to cope with a serious illness, a person and members of the family acquire specialized knowledge about disease and treatment. It is not unusual that children and adults with life-threatening or chronic illnesses acquire remarkable medical sophistication as they attempt to learn to live with their maladies. This helps them to maintain some control. It makes it possible for them to interact more effectively with those who care for them, and helps them to assume a partnership in medical efforts to treat their disease.

Persons with AIDS seek to understand the various illnesses that comprise this syndrome. Many struggle to learn ways to live with a disease for which there is, at present, no permanent cure. It is not uncommon that their experiences of a life-threatening illness dominate their conscious thoughts and conversation. A pastor needs basic factual knowledge about AIDS if he or she is to be able to interact effectively with infected persons who either have become sick or who fear they will get sick.

Much material has been published about AIDS since 1981 when Acquired Immunodeficiency Syndrome emerged as a major public health threat. The scientific literature adds approximately six hundred citations per month to an ever-increasing

1

data base of knowledge about AIDS. A significant amount of the scientific information filters into the popular press and other media. In this chapter we shall review some of these basic data on AIDS, not simply to reiterate the facts, but to draw out their importance for the pastoral care of persons with AIDS and their families.

AIDS Is Acquired

AIDS is an insidious disease, acquired during intimate sexual relations or in the exchange of blood. The principal route of infection is through sexual transmission. It is estimated that three-quarters of all AIDS-infected individuals in our country were exposed to the human immunodeficiency virus (HIV) while engaging in sexual activities.

AIDS is caused by a virus that is present in large amounts in certain body fluids, principally blood, semen, and vaginal secretions. The virus is transmitted when HIV particles or infected cells gain access to another person's bloodstream. This transfer can occur in a variety of ways including vaginal, anal, or oral-genital intercourse. It can likewise occur when the blood of an infectious person is intravenously transfused by sharing improperly sterilized needles. And finally, it can be passed on by an infected pregnant mother to an unborn or newborn child. Cases of infection by transfusion from contaminated blood have occurred. Since mid-1985 all donated blood is carefully screened for antibodies to the virus.

It is important to note that the disease is *acquired*. For some people this means that one is responsible for getting it. Unfortunately, large numbers of sexually active individuals and drug addicts were unknowingly exposed to HIV before much was known about the virus or how it is transmitted.

It is still uncertain how many individuals who have acquired the virus will eventually develop related symptoms (AIDS-related complex, ARC) or the full-blown clinical disease, AIDS. Although the odds for those infected with HIV range from 1-in-3 to 1-in-10 chances for developing the disease, the future clinical picture may be even more bleak. There is a potentially long interval between the time of infection and the appearance of symptoms. The incubation period may be between five and eight years or even longer. For this reason, pastors can appreciate the anxiety of many individuals who test positive for antibodies to the AIDS virus and who live with the ever-present fear that someday they will become sick and possibly die.

The probability of infection and disease may be related to a number of co-factors. Some have hypothesized that infection may be linked to the amount of the virus transmitted. Individuals engaged in high risk behaviors with multiple exposures may be at greater risk, for example, than a health care worker who has a single exposure to the virus through a needlestick injury with contaminated blood. Some individuals may be genetically more resistant to the virus than some others whose general health or body immunity may be compromised. On the other hand, a single exposure to the virus may be all that is required to become infected.

In an analogous way, a person who tests positive for AIDS antibodies may not develop symptoms. This may be related to general health and previous medical history, nutrition and exercise, environmental and economic variables, and a host of other related issues. Some others will develop symptoms rapidly and die soon after. Investigators are trying to understand the relationships among many of these co-factors that influence both infection and disease.

The link between behavioral choice and acquisition suggests why some individuals who have been exposed to the virus, or who go on to develop ARC or AIDS, experience feelings of culpability, blame, or guilt. Some feel responsible for getting the disease, or angry because they did not realize how vulnerable they were to acquiring the virus. The realization of infection or disease may serve as a catalyst for significant review of issues of lifestyle, choices, and responsibility.

A 30-year old man described his feelings about contracting AIDS in the following way: "I deserve to have gotten this thing. I've been a real whore for many years, and have been abusive to my body . . . I have no one but myself to thank for getting the big A."

While pastoral care should not focus on *how* or *why* a person has acquired the disease, the person with AIDS may need to identify and discuss these issues. Non-judgmental dialogue with the pastor can help a person to process effectively these feelings and concerns. We will return to this issue in another chapter when we discuss specific psychosocial concerns of persons with AIDS.

The Meaning of Immunodeficiency

AIDS is principally a disease of the body's immune system. The immune system functions to identify, isolate, and rid foreign invaders from the body. Since the role and functions of the human immune system are continually referenced when discussing AIDS, it seems useful to review some basic facts. Persons with AIDS, their families, and their health care providers speak knowledgeably about these issues. A pastor should also have a clear and working understanding of these basic biochemical issues. The following will provide a somewhat oversimplified picture of immune dysfunctioning and AIDS.

The human body's immune system is designed in such a way that it is virtually impenetrable by threatening organisms. This system relies on effective physical, chemical, and biochemical interactive barriers. The human immune system is made up of a variety of cells whose function is to identify and eliminate viruses, bacteria, and other foreign substances (antigens) from the body. Some of these foreign microorganisms have physical or chemical properties that make detection and destruction exceedingly difficult.

When the immune system recognizes a "foreigner" a number of specialized cells move into action. Many writers on the functioning of the human immune system utilize military language to describe the ways in which the body attempts to defend itself against foreign invaders. The armory of the human immune system is limited to several principal weapon systems. We shall briefly review these defensive systems since they are very relevant to our understanding of AIDS.

Phagocytes are one of these defensive weapons. As its Greek name suggests, phagocytes have the ability to "eat" invading viruses, bacteria, fungi, protozoa, or worms, as well as any other debris that washes into the bloodstream. These cells are largely scavengers, whose purpose is to clean up the body of any foreign material as well as dead tissue and degenerated cells. In the age of computer games, we have seen the work of phagocytes in the activities of PacMan, whose large mouth sets about the task of devouring any "enemy" in sight. This class of cells is non-specific, which means that they consume all kinds of cellular debris. The "big eaters" among these phagocytes are called macrophages. They play an indispensable role in immune system functioning.

Macrophages catalyze and potentiate the activities of almost every other cell of the immune system. Macrophages engage other helper cells. A specific subset of cells involved in these defensive immune functions are the white blood cells called lymphocytes. The lymphocytes are also patrolling the body, alert to foreign invaders. These circulating lymphocytes routinely attack infected cells and prevent the invading microorganisms from reproducing themselves and migrating to other sites.

A lymphocyte becomes a T-cell by passing through the thymus gland. That is how it acquires its name, T-cell. The specific function of the T-cell or "helper cell" is to coordinate and manage the activities of the immune system. A principal job performed by T-cells is to orchestrate immune response to an invading foreign microorganism. The T-cells stimulate the B-cells which produce specific antibodies that attack, neutralize or eliminate the invading virus or bacteria.

Some have described T-cells as the "watchdog" of the immune system, patrolling the body looking for potentially harmful foreign organisms. When it locates one of these organisms, it alerts the spleen and lymph nodes which in turn signal other T-cells in the body to reproduce and help fight the invader. When the infection is under control, the T-8, or suppressor cells call off the attack and the body returns to normal functioning.

As we know, viruses are incapable of independent life. A virus is nothing more than inert, organic material looking for a living cell in which it might reside. Only by invading a fully metabolized "host" cell can a virus become active, capable of reproducing its genetic material. A virus exploits the living cell which it invades. It uses the host cell's metabolic machinery to make many more virus particles which in time will seek out other host cells in order to perpetuate the process.

HIV, the human immunodeficiency virus associated with AIDS, directly attacks the T-helper cells by invading its structure, neutralizing its defenses, and rendering them ineffective. The T-cells are prevented from performing their infection-fighting functions. HIV can migrate freely within the body, proliferating within the T-cells it invades. The T-cells effectively become partners with the enemy, HIV.

When the HIV invades the T-4 cells, it becomes part of the cell's DNA, the molecular chain containing the genetic information enabling cells to reproduce. The virus can remain dormant for a considerable period of time, hence the long incubation period before a person manifests symptoms of AIDS. The only clear effect is that the T-4 cells cannot carry on their normal defensive functions.

When the HIV is activated, stimulated perhaps by some specific triggers, the virus does not waste any time reproducing itself and infecting other cells. Its genetic components allow it to replicate itself a thousand times faster than many other kinds of viruses. The T-cells in which HIV has made its home become "factories" in which the virus reproduces. The original host T-cells are killed in the process.

As the virus is released into the circulating blood it seeks out other T-cells, thus further debilitating the immune system and interrupting its important functions. The death of T-4 cells appears to precipitate immunological breakdown, and the symptoms of AIDS and ARC probably result from this event.

The immune system of a person infected with HIV attempts to fight the presence of the virus and produces antibodies. However, these antibodies appear to be ineffective in destroying the virus. With a decrease in the number of T-4 cells, the immune system is unable to discharge its important defensive and regulatory functions. The person who is immuno-compromised is thus unable to mount effective antibody reactions to new antigens, thus becoming vulnerable to a host of recurrent or new infections.

This very basic description of immunodeficiency resulting from exposure to HIV has symbolic relevance to pastoral care. An immunocompromised individual becomes defenseless. Immunodeficiency leaves a person feeling vulnerable, unprotected, under siege. The psychological and spiritual states of a person with AIDS frequently mirror the biological portrait of immunodeficiency. A person in this condition is vulnerable to subtle forms of rejection, real or perceived. An individual in a weakened physical state is prone to become disengaged, hopeless, and depressed, surrendering the will to fight, the will to live. While this is not a universal experience of persons with AIDS, the drama of human immunodeficiency can interpret the psychological and spiritual defenselessness some individuals feel.

The essential biological characteristics of this disease can precipitate a number of related negative psychological and spiritual reactions. A person who feels defenseless looks for someone who will be supportive. Pastoral care has the potential to be this much needed source of support.

AIDS Is a Syndrome

In contemporary medical usage, a syndrome describes an aggregate of symptoms associated with any disease. When all of these symptoms are put together, they form the clinical picture of the disease. Symptoms associated with AIDS or ARC include some of the following:

- persistent weariness
- chills and excessive nocturnal sweating
- significant weight loss (10% of normal body weight)
- swelling of lymph nodes (necks, armpit, groin)
- chronic diarrhea
- persistent dry cough
- white sore patches in mouth and throat (thrush)
- pink or purple blotches on or under skin

With a weakened immune system, an individual is prone to develop a variety of "opportunistic" infections which contribute to the clinical picture of this syndrome. The term "opportunistic" is used to describe a wide range of illnesses. These illnesses are attributable to organisms commonly present in the environment, but threatening only to persons whose immune systems have been weakened. These organisms use the "opportunity" provided by the body's compromised defenses to gain a firm foothold.

This is a unique characteristic of AIDS, namely that there is a tendency for an infected person to develop many problems, with the common denominator being suppression of normal immune functions. This makes medical management so difficult; the body is not able to assist effectively in dealing with infections and cancers. We can use the analogy of a dam with multiple leaks to exemplify the problem of AIDS management. While attention is being directed to plugging one leak, another hole springs open in the wall. Before long, there may be nine such holes, spread over the entire expanse of the dam, making effective containment a virtual impossibility.

Not only do the body's T-cells fail to fight off the HIV invader, but the other viruses living in check within the human body can express themselves in inimical ways as new forms of disease. Although the immune system is seriously impaired as a result of HIV infection, this does not mean that the individual is vulnerable to every infection. One of the characteristics of this syndrome is that the HIV infected individual appears to be particularly vulnerable to certain diseases. We would like to briefly identify and comment on the principal diseases associated with AIDS. In pastoral practice, these are the diseases one most commonly encounters.

Pneumocystis Carinii Pneumonia (PCP)

Among life-threatening opportunistic infections associated with immunodeficiency, Pneumocystis carinii pneumonia (PCP) is the most common. For a significant number of people, PCP is the first manifestation of AIDS.

PCP is caused by an infection of the lungs by a single-celled parasite (protozoan). The parasite, Pneumocystis carinii, has been found in the lungs of animals and healthy humans. Although present, it does not flourish unless the immune system is significantly weakened. If the parasite is activated, it multiplies and consolidates the air spaces in the lungs in a honeycomb-like fashion. The initial manifestations of this disease are common to other forms of pneumonia: dry cough, fever, and breathing problems. A thirty-three-year old man who had been ill for some time before he got PCP described the pneumonia:

> *I felt lousy for a couple of weeks, but thought it was just a common winter flu. My energy was like zero. . . . It was a struggle walking from my apartment to the store and back. I was running a fever, and felt terrible. Breathing was labored; I was literally gasping for breath. It scared me so much that I finally called a friend who helped me get over to the emergency room at the hospital.*

Since AIDS is a syndrome, it is not uncommon that a single individual may develop several major infections and cancers. PCP occurs at least once in about three-quarters of persons with AIDS. Improved treatment and maintenance programs have increased survival rates for those who develop PCP. The pneumonia is responsive to a variety of antibiotic and other drug treatments. The sulfa drugs used in the management of PCP, especially Bactrim and Septra, often have unpleasant side-effects, including rash and fever.

Even though an individual may respond well to treatment, the possibility of recurrent infection is high, because the immune system does not appear to recover. If the immunosuppression reversed, the infection would be checked in its progress. With each successive bout of PCP, however, an individual's chances for survival are decreased. Overall mortality rates for this infection have remained relatively constant since PCP began to be monitored in 1981, and PCP continues to be the major cause of death in persons with AIDS.

Kaposi's Sarcoma (KS)

Before its manifestation in persons with AIDS, Kaposi's sarcoma (KS) was seen clinically in older men. Kaposi's sarcoma is a cancer originating from the cells of the walls of the small blood vessels. It is not a new cancer, but is recorded in the annals of medicine more than a hundred years ago. The cancer carries the name of Moricz Kaposi, a Hungarian physician, who reported slow-growing tumors in a population of elderly men.

Apart from its association with AIDS, the cancer is not life-threatening. The cancer produces slowly developing lesions on body surfaces. Ordinarily, these cancerous lesions remain localized, usually on the leg, and do not spread to other parts of the body.

With the advent of AIDS, this rare form of cancer began appearing in the population of homosexual men infected with the HIV virus. Unlike the form of KS seen in people without AIDS, the cancer is widely disseminated in persons with AIDS. In this latter group the cancer is more aggressive than in earlier clinical descriptions. The lesions are not restricted to the legs of a patient, but may appear anywhere on the body. When associated with AIDS, these blotches commonly appear on the skin of the feet, the trunk of the body, on the head, neck, face, eyes, mouth, and throat. Lesions can also appear in the internal organs, such as in the gastrointestinal tract as well as on the lymph nodes.

The cancer is first visible when painless purple to brown colored, flat or raised, irregularly shaped blotches appear on or under the skin. Initially they look like ordinary bruise marks, but they do not disappear after a week or so. The lesions frequently are raised above the level of the surrounding skin and are hard to the touch.

Kaposi's sarcoma is rarely the primary cause of death for a person with AIDS. If the cancer appears in the throat or other internal organs, the threat to life increases. The treatments for these lesions with radiation and chemotherapies can be effective, but they can further suppress the immune system to such a degree that the treatments for KS may pave the way for other opportunistic infections.

From a pastoral perspective, the disfigurement associated with this cancer, particularly on exposed skin surfaces like the face, neck, upper torso, and limbs, can cause psychological distress for the person. The proliferation of lesions can disturb individuals who interact with KS patients, and may become an obstacle to effective pastoral care.

John was forty-nine years old and was being treated in hospital for a primary PCP infection; he was also being treated for rapidly spreading KS which covered the surface tissue of his face, neck, and arms. He had lost approximately forty pounds of body weight during the past three months. Emaciated and weak, yet alert and interactive, he asked to receive the sacrament of the sick as a Roman Catholic. Because he was coughing considerably, the hospital required full precautions, including mask.

A priest, inexperienced in providing pastoral care to persons with AIDS, was called from a nearby parish to minister to John. When he arrived at the hospital and identified himself at the nursing station, he was informed about the precautions.

After a brief introduction, the priest proceeded to administer the sacrament of the sick, nervously performing the anointing using surgical gloves. After the rite was completed, it was clear that the priest wanted to make a hasty retreat. John, however, detained him a bit. He thanked him for coming, but asked him if he were afraid he might catch the disease if he touched his forehead disfigured with extensive KS lesions. The priest defensively said, "Of course not, but the hospital staff insists I protect myself."

In a situation like this, would direct human contact in the ritual acts of imposition of hands and anointing have brought greater comfort and reassurance to this seriously ill man? Might those gestures have spoken of greater acceptance and support had they been performed in a context of open acknowledgement and comfort with the physical condition of the person with AIDS? These are issues which will be explored later when we turn our attention to psychosocial concerns.

Cytomegalovirus (CMV)

There are other diseases associated with AIDS. Some of these involve parasitic infections, yeast infections, fungal and bacterial infections. However, the viral infection which is most life-threatening to a person with AIDS is Cytomegalovirus, commonly called CMV. Evidence of CMV infection is almost universal in homosexual men with AIDS, and it is common in others presenting with the syndrome. It is suspected that CMV plays a role in the development of Kaposi's sarcoma. The infection contributes to blindness, seizures and dementia, pneumonia, inflammation of the esophagus, and pernicious diarrhea.

Infection with CMV is common in a large percentage of adults. However, the virus remains latent in the body for long periods. When it does become active in otherwise healthy persons, it produces a variety of symptoms ranging from skin rash to a mononucleosis-type syndrome. If the virus reactivates during a woman's pregnancy, it can infect the fetus, contributing to congenital defects including mental retardation. Like other slow viruses, the reasons why the dormant virus reactivates are not known.

In the early years of the AIDS pandemic, if there was a single picture of a person with AIDS dying a slow, painful, wasting death, it was usually associated with CMV. Now there are new drugs that interrupt the CMV from replicating, which assist in medical management of the person with this viral infection.

Barbara Peabody has published a journal, *The Screaming Room,* documenting her memories and feelings as she provided principal care for her twenty-nine year old son, Peter, during his terminal illness. Peter was an example of a person with AIDS whose primary infection and cause of death was CMV. It explained his blindness, vertigo, paralysis, cerebral and neurological changes, and the final pneumonia which eventually claimed his life.

Peter's story—told through his mother's journal—of his eleven-month battle with AIDS is not atypical of many others with CMV. Peter received numerous antiviral drugs, and had short periods of improvement. But his story was one of multiple relapses, uncontrollable diarrhea, and unpredictable seizures. In words recorded as epilogue to her journal she writes: "As I read the results [of the autopsy], I wondered for the thousandth time how Peter endured such overwhelming physical devastation for so long, wondered at the fortitude and unwavering hope that turned him from boy to man."

Toxoplasmosis

One of the more distressing management issues in the care of a person with AIDS is when the disease dramatically affects higher brain functioning. Toxoplasmosis is one of the most common causes of central nervous system disease among persons with AIDS. It is a principal agent in altering cognitive and language abilities. This parasite, *Toxoplasma gondii*, invades the central nervous system, triggering brain seizures, high fevers and delirium, and decreases levels of consciousness. Personality and behavior changes associated with this brain infection are often the most disturbing aspects of this disease. Family members and those caring for an individual infected with *Toxoplasma gondii* report difficulty in coping with these alterations in personality. The part of the brain controlling speech is also affected. Some persons infected with this parasite become unable to speak.

The infection is one of the most effectively treatable AIDS-related opportunistic infections. People with toxoplasmosis respond promptly to drug therapy. However, the infection is likely to recur unless medication is continued on a maintenance program. As in other infections, the long-term use of such drugs can have many undesirable side-effects, and can do additional damage to the immune system. The image evoked earlier of the finger in the dam is an apt description of the problem associated with the medical management of many AIDS-related infections.

Cryptosporidiosis

Cryptosporidiosis is a parasitic infection, virtually unknown in humans prior to the advent of AIDS in the early 1980s. The parasite, *Cryptosporidium difficile,* had been found in a number of animals and reptiles, but rarely in human persons. In the few human cases in which the parasite had been documented, the diarrhea resulting from infection was self-limiting. This is not the case when the parasite attacks a person with AIDS. The diarrhea is sustained and life-threatening. This pernicious diarrhea results in a person being unable to absorb nutrients from food, contributing to severe loss of weight, dehydration, and malnutrition.

Because the parasite is found particularly in animal, bird, and reptile fecal materials, persons with AIDS need to exercise care when exposed to these potential sources of infection. Barbara Peabody, in *The Screaming Room*, recalls her son's fear of infection from this source.

> *"I hope they don't fly in here," Peter says, standing by the window and watching two pigeons on the concrete ledge outside. The ledge is covered with white pigeon droppings. He has an obsessive fear of animals and the germs they could give him. He cringes when the neighbors' terrier bounds into our house for a minute and is afraid of the aviary around the patio at John's house. Though all the birds are caged, he insists that they get loose and are in the thickly-twined branches shading the patio, that their feather dust or droppings could fall on him.*
>
> *"Maybe we should close the window," he suggests.*
>
> *"I don't think they can get in, Peter; it only opens about five inches, and it gets so stuffy in here without air-conditioning."*
>
> *"Well, I think they could," he says, eyeing the window suspiciously as he crawls back into bed. "Lower it a little bit."*
>
> *"Okay, a little," I agree, narrowing the opening to three inches. He continues glancing apprehensively at the window, then dozes off.*
>
> (The Screaming Room, p. 94)

Although there have been a number of drugs used to treat the cryptosporidium parasitic infection, these have not proven to be effective in controlled human trials. The best that medications have been able to achieve is a reduction in discomfort associated with persistent diarrhea.

Mycobacterium Avium-Intracellular (MAI)

The bacterium, MAI, is commonly found in the environment, for example in dust, soil, water. Despite its ubiquity, it rarely causes disease in humans, except in those who are immune compromised. When the bacteria takes hold in a person with a weakened immune system, the lungs are usually affected. In persons with AIDS, the infection will frequently spread to the liver, spleen, lymph nodes, gastrointestinal tract, bone marrow, and brain.

The associated symptoms of MAI are similar to other AIDS-related diseases: fever, weight loss, cough, respiratory distress, swollen lymph glands, abdominal cramping and diarrhea.

MAI is resistant to standard antituberculosis drugs, although some new experimental drugs are promising.

AIDS-Related Complex (ARC)

There are numerous cases of individuals who have been exposed to HIV, but do not develop the full spectrum of related illnesses, some of which are described above and which constitute a diagnosis of AIDS. AIDS-related complex or ARC describes those individuals whose symptoms stem from the HIV infection but do not meet the specific diagnostic criteria of the Centers for Disease Control for AIDS. ARC is not as well defined as is the full clinical syndrome, AIDS, although many of the symptoms parallel those of AIDS.

A person with ARC usually presents with symptoms including fatigue, low energy level, significant weight loss associated with anemia, diarrhea, oral yeast infections, petechiae or bruising, swollen glands in groin, neck, or underarms, nocturnal sweating, rashes, chills, and fever. Clinically, the blood profile of a person with ARC will reveal low T-4-cell numbers, a higher ratio of T-8 (suppressor) to T-4 (helper) cells, and other manifestations of immunodeficient functioning. Persons with ARC present a full range of neuropsychological symptoms directly associated with the HIV infection. Brain dysfunctions, including cognitive impairment, memory loss, perceptual problems, seizures, paralysis, and personality changes are common in more than half of all persons with AIDS or ARC.

There may be more than a quarter of a million people in the United States today with ARC. Some may go on to develop AIDS; others may not progress. The question foremost in the minds of persons with ARC is: "Will I get AIDS?" It is difficult to estimate how many individuals with ARC will progress to a full diagnosis of AIDS. A significant number of persons with ARC will die from these related diseases without a diagnosis of AIDS.

Persons with ARC not only have a number of physical problems with which to contend, but also share the persistent feeling of insecurity about their futures. Not knowing how the virus will impact their future morbidity and mortality is psychologically disabling for many persons. They feel that they live their lives perilously positioned under the sword of Damocles, wondering when the hair will snap and the sword will fall.

Pastoral Implications

We have begun our discussion of Acquired Immunodeficiency Syndrome with a survey of some of the basic clinical facts. These basic issues help us to understand better the physical and emotional experiences of persons with AIDS and ARC, or who are HIV antibody positive. Pastors may debate the necessity of knowing these clinical details. It is our position that the pastoral care of persons with AIDS is enhanced when the pastor appreciates the physical, psychological, and social concerns they share. For these reasons, it is important that pastors stay current as new knowledge about AIDS and its treatment are published. We may conceptualize pastoral care as an essentially spiritual ministry. However, our efforts are enhanced to the degree we understand the collateral concerns of the persons to whom we minister.

In the remainder of this book we shall presume on this basic understanding of what AIDS is and how it affects the physical, psychological, social, and spiritual functioning of persons affected. As pastors we need to think about AIDS holistically. Our strategies for pastoral care hinge on how able we are to integrate effectively our knowledge about this new disease with our other experiences in ministering to persons with life-threatening illnesses.

2

Engaging in Pastoral Care
with Persons with AIDS

In the natural history of medicine, AIDS is without effective parallel. It is a disease that has exposed some of the flaws in our social fabric. Having a severely stigmatizing disease, persons with AIDS fear discovery, discrimination, rejection, and abandonment. The social and psychological stresses that compound the physical characteristics of AIDS are significant, and effective management of these problems challenges all providers of care. In this chapter we shall consider some of the specific problems which pastors encounter in ministering to persons with AIDS and the significant others (spouse, parent, child, sibling, lover, friend) who are their primary care givers.

Dealing with One's Own
Attitudes Toward AIDS

There are many experiences in human life that serve as catalysts for questioning, reflection, and personal growth. In routine pastoral practice, continually we are confronted with human struggles that demand examination of our thoughts, feelings, biases, prejudices, and fears. Pastoral care requires continual engagement with personal values, religious beliefs, and theologies.

Involvement in the pastoral care of persons with AIDS raises its own particular set of questions. Let's review some of

17

the attitudes that pastors and others who choose to care for persons with AIDS need to consider.

AIDS: The Disease

As noted in the opening chapter, the best medical knowledge affirms that AIDS is a disease that is principally transmitted either sexually or with IV needles. Unlike other life-threatening illnesses, persons infected with the AIDS virus or who develop symptoms related to the syndrome, experience stigma. Persons with AIDS are not the only ones affected by social response to the disease; those individuals who become involved in providing care likewise are vulnerable to the negative reactions of others. It is important to acknowledge this social reality before embarking on a decision to assume a helping role in the care of a person with AIDS.

Doctors and nurses who care for persons with AIDS report the negative comments of some of their colleagues. Some report that some physicians stop referring new patients to colleagues who are known to have AIDS patients in their practice. Despite clear and factual evidence concerning the transmission of the virus associated with AIDS, some individuals are still anxious about becoming infected through casual contact.

Some pastors, along with health care professionals, have reported the objections of their spouses to their involvements with persons with AIDS. The medical literature is becoming more involved with ethical issues pertaining to care of persons with AIDS. Specifically, are physicians ethically obliged to care for someone with AIDS? It is interesting to note that fear of infection, while certainly one area of concern, is not the most salient reason for physicians' reticence to become involved in AIDS patient care. We will return to some of the other reasons that interpret their reluctance later in this chapter.

It is crucial, nonetheless, for a pastor to reconcile any fears about becoming infected through contacts in ordinary pastoral care. AIDS is a difficult disease to get. AIDS education continually stresses that an individual cannot get the disease by touching, kissing, or embracing someone, or sharing a communion cup. You cannot get it from a person coughing or sneezing on you. We are told that the disease is transmitted only one way: when the semen, vaginal secretions or blood of a person infected with the AIDS virus directly enters the bloodstream of someone who is not infected. Despite the strong evidence about how the virus is and is not transmitted, fears of infection can still exist among individuals exposed to persons with AIDS.

A parishioner had been hospitalized twice in the course of four months for AIDS-related opportunistic infections. Hearing rumors from others within the parish that Fred Thompson had contracted AIDS, the pastor resisted visitation during the period of Fred's convalescence after his discharge from the hospital. Fred was a fifty-two year old married man. His wife, Beth, was providing principal care for her husband at home. When his disease progressed, he was readmitted to the hospital. The family had been members of the parish for many years, although their participation in the parochial community was minimal.

Distraught by the absence of the pastor during the previous four months of crisis, the wife made an appointment and visited with her pastor. In the course of her visit she shared with the pastor some of the important details about her husband's diagnosis and his present medical crisis. She asked him specifically if he would pay a call on her husband in the hospital. The pastor hesitantly agreed that he would.

Two days later the visit took place. When the pastor entered Fred's room he stood very close to the door and spoke to Fred from that position. He never approached the bed. The visit was awkward. Although the pastor knew that Fred's condition was rapidly deteriorating and that death was probable, he was not able to address these realities. His conversation tended to become a monologue in which he exhorted Fred to maintain his courage, his faith, and his will to overcome this disease. Fred was silently unresponsive to the pastor's communication. After offering a hasty prayer, the pastor quickly departed.

The pastor's behavior in this case is best explained in terms of irrational fears and anxieties associated with the disease. It is understandable that people harbor legitimate fears about a disease as lethal as AIDS. However, those fears can affect the ability to minister to persons who need pastoral support. More importantly, a pastor's irrational fears can cause additional pain and harm to persons with AIDS and those who attempt to care for them. In the case cited above, it is easy to understand and forgive the pastor's inappropriate behavior. Understanding and forgiveness, however, do not mitigate the injury Fred and his wife experienced as a result of the pastor's fears.

Feelings Toward Persons with AIDS

As the number of cases of AIDS began to increase in the early 1980s, the media began slowly to report the facts concerning this emerging social and public health problem. In reviewing the short history of this disease, some social scientists have hypothesized that the general public, the media, and federal, state, and local governments resisted seeing AIDS as a major health problem until non-stigmatized groups became concerned about their own susceptibility.

During the first year of its identified existence, AIDS was primarily associated with homosexual men. For a brief time, predating the labeling of the disease as Acquired Immunodeficiency Syndrome, the disease was described as Gay-Related Immune Deficiency, GRID. This designation was introduced despite the fact that there were increasing numbers of reported cases of the disease among non-homosexual populations including drug users, Haitians, and hemophiliacs. The media and government became more engaged when AIDS was diagnosed in children, resulting from virus-contaminated transfusions or prenatal transmission from infected mothers. Despite the realization that the disease has little regard for age, gender, or sexual preference, it has been difficult altering a popular notion that AIDS is considered a "gay disease."

We have previously acknowledged the resistance of some physicians to become involved in the care of persons with AIDS. One cause for this resistance is the dislike or discomfort with persons in certain high-risk groups who develop the disease. Although there are other "at risk" groups in addition to gay men and IV drug users, these latter groups still account for approximately three-quarters of reported cases.

Some physicians have acknowledged that they dislike caring for gay men and IV drug users. It is not uncommon that physicians have little empathy for persons whom they characterize as contracting AIDS through self-inflicted exposure and infection. It would be inaccurate to conclude that a significant number of physicians harbor hostile feelings toward persons with AIDS, but unconscious feelings can color decisions about initiating care and the quality of care provided.

In any helping relationship, it is important for the helper to pay attention to feelings he or she experiences toward the person seeking assistance. It is difficult to be effective in a helping relationship if one has strong negative feelings and judgments toward the individual seeking help. To attempt to provide care without attending to and resolving personal issues related to the individual is irresponsible. Sometimes helpers create more problems for the helpee than they solve. In medicine, these problems are termed iatrogenic, meaning they have their origin in the attitudes and behaviors of physicians toward their patients.

The same phenomenon can exist in pastoral care, when a pastor's overt or covert hostility or negative attitudes can intensify a person's suffering. The following story of one bishop's pastoral care for a priest who was dying of AIDS underscores a positive, accepting approach.

In April 1987, Archbishop James Hickey, of the Roman Catholic Archdiocese of Washington, D.C., in an unprecedented statement, revealed that forty-four year old Fr. Michael Peterson had died of AIDS. Peterson, a psychiatrist and director of Saint Luke's Institute for the treatment of drug and sexual dependencies in priests and religious women and men, died within a year of his diagnosis.

The focus of Archbishop Hickey's pastoral care for Father Peterson in his struggle with AIDS is reflected in the archbishop's statement at the time of Peterson's death. "His tragic death is a reminder to us of the personal and human dimensions of this growing epidemic," he remarked. A month before his death, Archbishop Hickey encouraged Father Peterson to write to all the priests of the Archdiocese of Washington and to bishops across the United States who had referred priests and religious to Saint Luke's Institute. The archbishop was sensitive to the isolation that a person with AIDS can feel, and took deliberate steps to help Father Peterson realize the understanding, acceptance, and support of his associates in the ministry.

It is also clear from the archbishop's public statement that he was not threatened by the implications of how Father Peterson may have contracted the deadly virus. He acknowledged that he did not know how the priest had become infected, and that this was not relevant. The archbishop said: "What is most important is not how he died, but how he served." Hickey's sole concern, in his own words, was "to reach out with support, prayers, and assistance, as his bishop, as his friend and his brother in the Lord."

In joint pastoral letters Catholic bishops throughout the United States are taking leadership in pointing out not only the necessity of providing pastoral assistance to persons with AIDS and to those who care for them, but also for tolerance. The focus of their exhortations is directed to the antipathies some clergy may feel toward persons in the high-risk AIDS populations.

The California bishops in their April 1987 letter entitled "A Call to Compassion" urged their people to treat those suffering with AIDS with care and compassion, not judgment. Recalling that Jesus healed "the outcasts and the wounded of his world" the bishops suggested that the Catholic Church should imitate this behavior and care for those who have AIDS "without judging or imputing blame." Interpreting the traditional mission of the Church, the bishops described Catholics as "disciples of Jesus Christ," whose mandate is to "care for the sick, to show them they are loved." They described persons with AIDS as "sisters and brothers of Jesus (who) bear a special resemblance to him because of their suffering." The bishops said: "People with AIDS-ARC remind us that they are not distant and unfamiliar victims to be pitied or shunned, but persons who deserve to remain within our communal consciousness and to be embraced with unconditional love."

In June 1987 the Catholic bishops of New Jersey issued a policy statement on AIDS commenting on four primary relationships of the Church to individuals with the virus: pastoral minister, employer, educator, and social service provider. The bishops acknowledged at the beginning of their policy statement that "the growing AIDS crisis requires a compassionate response." Focusing on the principal relationship of the Church as pastor to persons with AIDS, the bishops recognized their obligation to provide pastoral ministry to their sisters and brothers "at every stage in the disease's progression, and to their families, friends, and associates." The bishops want to insure that all those who minister to persons with AIDS have appropriate training and work in collaboration with other appropriate agencies. Recognizing the potential strain or burnout on those providing such ministry to persons with AIDS, the bishops have mandated that support networks be established to assist pastors.

The policy statement, governing pastoral care of Catholics in the New Jersey dioceses, clearly states that "persons with AIDS shall have the rights to the sacraments and Christian burial," and that the identity of such a person is confidential and "every precaution shall be taken by a pastoral minister to maintain that confidentiality." The Church, in developing these guidelines, acknowledges the implicit stigma that many persons with AIDS have felt. Many have experienced alienation from the Church prior to becoming ill. In addressing the issues of incorporation (access to sacraments and Christian burial) and the right to confidentiality, the bishops have taken a positive and constructive step toward achieving the desired compassion and reconciliation that are the bedrock of all effective pastoral ministry.

Pastors and physicians share parallel responsibilities in relation to the provision of care for persons with AIDS. Society presumes that doctors and clergy will provide care for all persons. In return for the special status that society accords physical and spiritual healers, it expects its physicians and pastors to be self-sacrificing. In December 1986, in a statement on AIDS reported by the Council of Ethical and Judicial Affairs of the American Medical Association, the following position was articulated. Acknowledging medicine's tradition of providing care to infectious persons, the AMA said that "not everyone is emotionally able to care for patients with AIDS."

Not every pastor is emotionally able to care for a person with AIDS. It is important to reconcile this fact and make other provisions for the person's care. We would rarely encounter a situation where a pastor overtly would refuse ministerial assistance to a person with AIDS. To do so would be scandalous and unacceptable behavior, not in keeping with one's public profession. What is more disturbing, however, is covert refusal.

The case of Fred Thompson cited above exemplifies this point. The pastor's wife, knowing the alleged circumstances surrounding Thompson's diagnosis, was opposed to her husband's involvement in the case. The pastor himself was ambivalent, and his wife's fears effectively obstructed his ability to provide pastoral assistance to the Thompsons.

The pastor's expressed intentions were that he should get over to see Fred and Beth, but he never seemed to find the time in his schedule to accomplish his plan. He reasoned that if Fred wanted to see him, he would call. He thought that Fred probably was receiving adequate pastoral care from the chaplains connected with the VA hospital where he had been a patient. In all of these rationalizations, what is at issue is that the pastor perhaps is unable to provide effective care for a person with AIDS. If there are issues which are remediable, the pastor needs to deal with them. If, on the other hand, the barriers are not easily penetrable, then he or she needs to acknowledge the inability and make specific arrangements for referral to another person who is able to minister effectively to the family.

Confronting Personal Mortality

The majority of persons with AIDS for whom we care as pastors are young men and women. Many of these afflicted persons profess a valiant commitment to live despite the disabling aspects of AIDS. Yet for all of these individuals, the disease proves to be a terminal illness. Their trajectories to death may be either slow or accelerated, but eventually all die.

People in the health care professions who provide care for persons with AIDS speak about their frustration in seeing so many promising young people become ill, progressively deteriorate, and ultimately die. These physicians, nurses, and other care providers become very involved with persons with AIDS and with their families and friends. The person with AIDS becomes a first priority concern. Inevitably bonding takes place. Where there is attachment, there will be experiences of loss and grief when the person dies. We will discuss this point in detail in a subsequent chapter.

Health care providers not only describe their subjective experiences of burnout from working so hard to manage the multiple physical and emotional problems of persons with AIDS, but they also acknowledge the cumulative effect of working with so many people who die. Although they are dedicated to this work, a number of individuals find that they have to leave work with persons with AIDS because the confrontation with death proves to be too strong.

Chronic illness necessarily raises the issues of personal mortality. It is extremely difficult to imagine ourselves as dead. Dr. Elisabeth Kübler-Ross in her workshops on death and dying issues with hospital personnel has frequently commented that many of us perpetuate the illusion, "And thou and thou, but never me." It is an understandable defense. Dying persons, however, have a way of eroding the thin protective barrier, and make us come to terms with our personal mortality.

Dealing with the Experiences
of Persons with AIDS

AIDS has been experienced as a frontal attack on the death-denying character of our American culture. As a people we take every opportunity to shield ourselves from the realities of death. Our customs prefer to see individuals die in hospitals or nursing homes, away from the comfort and security of their own homes, surrounded by family members. The hospice movement, assisting terminally ill persons to die in the more natural context of their home and with the direct support of family members, is a somewhat countercultural phenomenon. It is not that American society is inhumane in dealing with dying persons; however, the American way of death underscores how uncomfortable we are with death.

The realities of AIDS are attacking the frontiers of the American consciousness about death. A life-threatening syndrome of diseases of incalculable proportion, AIDS is piercing the thin sheathing that protects a vulnerable nerve from unwanted stimulation. Continually we are confronted with statistics and projections about this epidemic. It is discomforting to learn that by the year 1991, it is anticipated that there will be a cumulative total of cases of AIDS in the United States in excess of a quarter of a million. Of that number approximately 180,000 people will have died by the end of that year. The vast majority of these cases will continue to come from the currently recognized high-risk groups, homosexual men and intravenous drug users, although there will be significant increases in the number of heterosexual and pediatric AIDS cases. Because of the large number of people who already are presumed to be infected with HIV, it is not anticipated that the reported rate of increase in AIDS cases will soon reverse itself. Into the next century, America will have to face the reality that deaths resulting from HIV infections will continue to rise.

It is with this escalating medical and psychological crisis in mind that health care is preparing itself in order effectively to meet new challenges to provide counsel and care. It is within this same context that those involved in pastoral ministries within the churches and synagogues must prepare for the new demands they will inevitably encounter in increasing numbers.

In the remainder of this chapter we shall consider the place of denial and anger in experiences of persons with AIDS. Pastors frequently encounter these two defenses in work with persons with life-threatening illnesses. Denial and anger have particular relevance in pastoral care with persons with AIDS.

Denial

Healthy psychological functioning depends upon the effective use of defense mechanisms. The principal purpose of psychological defenses is to assist a person to meet the challenges presented by a specific crisis. During a person's lifetime, a pattern of useful defenses and how they are employed is defined.

Denial is one of the more common of these unconscious defenses. By unconscious, we simply mean that a person is not aware that he or she is using this defense to cope with a particular threat. Denial protects a person in the face of facts and consequences that one is unwilling or otherwise unprepared to face. Denial is a complex mental mechanism that has a vital relationship to healthy adjustment and adaptation. For many persons denial may be quite functional.

It takes time to assimilate the facts and consequences about one's condition, especially when the information is that one has AIDS. It is understandable that a person may resist the medical conclusion, may plead diagnostic error, may dispute the prognosis offered. Some physicians may become embroiled in a debate with a patient over the medical facts. Effectively, the physician is attacking the psychological defense upon which the patient is relying in order to begin to cope with the news. A better strategy is to allow the patient to remain secure in his or her denial. After a while, denial often gives way to acceptance.

In healthy individuals, denial is a temporary solution, not a permanent one. It is a transitional state, a bridge between the world as it is and the world as we would like it to be. Occasionally, an individual rigidly clings to denial, and sometimes dies still maintaining that he or she is not seriously ill. The majority of people utilize denial as a temporary retreat while they better prepare themselves for engagement with the facts and consequences of their illness.

Some pastors experience difficulty in dealing with persons who are denying the facts of their situation. However, it is important to underscore the appropriateness, normality, and, for a number of people, the necessity of denial. Denial may resurface a number of times in the course of ministering to a person with AIDS, and to those who are their loved ones and care-providers.

One pastor reported the following case where she experienced distress in dealing with a person who was expressing significant denial.

Marc was a thirty-two year old musician. He played French horn in a symphonic orchestra in the city, and was a member of a chamber group as well. Marc also had a long history of intravenous drug use. He was first diagnosed with ARC, manifested in his case by persistent lymphadenopathy, prolonged swelling of the lymph nodes in his neck, armpits, and groin. His physician was diligent in his efforts to help Marc understand what the diagnosis of ARC meant, and to counsel him on strategies for health maintenance and the avoidance of high-risk behaviors. Although Marc was stunned to learn of his condition, he did not believe that he would progress on to AIDS. He believed that he was a strong and healthy person, from a family with a history of longevity, and that he would beat this disease.

Eight months later when he developed initial Kaposi's sarcoma lesions on his chest, he avoided bringing them to the attention of his physician for an additional three months. As they further developed in size and intensity of color, he reluctantly disclosed their presence to his doctor. When he was seen by his physician in relation to the lesions, it was discovered that the KS had infected his lungs. The doctor's prognosis was that he would probably live about two or three months.

Marc was unwilling to accept this information, and protested that he would prove the doctors wrong. His attending physician did not attempt to argue with his denial. When the hospital chaplain visited him, she sensitively attempted to explore his willingness to talk about his diagnosis and his feelings.

Marc was a gregarious and self-assured person. His personal manner was engaging. Marc was responsive to the chaplain, but did not pick up on any opening the chaplain provided him to explore his feelings related to his pulmonary diagnosis. He called his lung problems "minor" and assured her that he would be out of the hospital in no time, and back to work with the orchestra.

Marc remained hospitalized for fifty-eight days until his death. During that time, as his physical condition deteriorated, the chaplain continued to visit him and attempted to assist him. He continued to maintain his denial, and she was frustrated that she was unable to break through to him. In reflecting and commenting on this experience, she noted two things. First, she realized that she had become attached to Marc during his terminal illness and had become a confederate in his denial. Second, she felt that she had failed him because she was unable to get him to prepare for death since he never acknowledged that he was terminally ill. After Marc's death, the chaplain experienced a mixture of feelings: satisfaction in the relationship she was able to establish with him, and failure in her inability to help him to move from his rigid denial.

Denial operates in other ways as well. A person can reject treatments and dispense with taking prescribed medications.

Because an individual does not accept the seriousness of his or her illness, he or she can engage in injurious behaviors, including excessive drinking and other forms of substance abuse. The person may not monitor diet and sleep habits, adding further stress to the body's ability to fight infection. If the individual is sexually active, he or she may continue to expose others to infection through unsafe practices.

A widowed mother whose twenty-four year old son was diagnosed with AIDS sought the counsel of her pastor. Having been raised in a strong Roman Catholic family, this woman looked to the priest as a trusted confidant and friend. Her son had Kaposi's sarcoma lesions on his leg, but with no other evidence of opportunistic infections. Since he was relatively healthy, he continued to live with a lover in Boston.

Distraught by the double news of his homosexual lifestyle and his infection with AIDS, the mother sought pastoral counseling with the pastor of her local parish. The priest knew the family well, and had known Paul when he was still living with the family. Since Paul had moved to Boston, the priest had only occasional contact with him. Paul had never discussed his lifestyle or his diagnosis with the pastor.

Mrs. Sheehan was concerned because she received a call from Paul's lover, Jonathan. Although she had never met Jonathan, recently she had become aware of their relationship. Paul and Jonathan had been together for about eight months at the time of Paul's diagnosis and they chose to continue their relationship. Reluctantly, Jonathan called Mrs. Sheehan because he was alarmed by Paul's behavior. In desperation he sought assistance.

Jonathan was concerned that Paul was acting in what he termed "self-destructive" ways. Paul's behavior was upsetting their relationship to the point where Jonathan was close to pulling away. Paul was drinking excessively, spending many nights in after-hours bars. He was losing weight, and was looking haggard. Jonathan tried to confront him about this, reminding him that he has AIDS and must be extremely vigilant. Paul says: "If I'm going to die, I'm going to die." In Jonathan's words: "Mrs. Sheehan, he acts as if he doesn't believe he's sick."

Mrs. Sheehan brought this problem to her pastor, asking him to help her decide what she should do, and how best to intervene with Paul. She had promised Jonathan that definitely she would do something. The pastor was uncertain what to advise. He admitted that his intuition was that Paul needed to be confronted, not only because he was compromising further his own physical health, but because he was potentially endangering others by his alleged risky sexual behaviors outside his relationship with Jonathan.

Mrs. Sheehan had interpreted Jonathan's concerns to mean that Paul not only was drinking a lot, but that he was irresponsibly promiscuous. The pastor felt among the family members and friends that Mrs. Sheehan had the closest relationship to her son. His counsel, therefore, was that with the assistance of a social worker or counselor from the AIDS Action Coalition in Boston, she visit Paul and begin to help him to accept the reality of his diagnosis. The pastor helped her to make the necessary contacts, and continued his personal support for her.

Denial can be employed by family or friends as well. Admittedly, it is difficult to acknowledge that someone you love is seriously ill and will die. It is a fine line to walk between continuing to treat a person with AIDS as alive, while also recognizing and adjusting to the reality that the person is dying as a result of this disease. Denial sometimes prevents the latter task from taking place.

There are situations in which a person with AIDS, who is aware and accepting of the reality of his or her diagnosis, is faced with family, lover, or friends who are unwilling to accept the same reality. In essence denial functions as a psychological block preventing open awareness of the life-threatening diagnosis and acceptance of the fact of death. By their words and behavior, others pretend that the evidence of the disease is not compelling, and that the person with AIDS will be able to conquer the illness. This pretense is different from a realistic attitude of hope and the desire to live which will be discussed fully in another chapter.

Living with a life-threatening illness requires that the person with AIDS and those who are important members of his or her support network be able to experience the feelings which are catalyzed by the illness. Together they need to experience the losses which are a natural part of this process, and be able to talk freely as the time of death draws closer. If a person with AIDS is to engage positively in this process, he or she must feel support and acceptance from those who share this experience. If that support and acceptance is not perceived, then the person with AIDS may feel isolated and vulnerable to fears of being abandoned.

Some pastors, in efforts to express positive support and to stimulate hope, become confederates in denial. They either pretend that the person is not as sick as he or she truly is, or they become allies with the denial of some important members of the family.

Susan was a twenty-six year old single mother who from her late teen years had been living independently of her family. Her son, Todd, was three years old. Susan, an IV-drug user, was diagnosed with Pneumocystis and was hospitalized. Her mother, Anne Stapleton, assumed care for Todd.

The relationship between Susan and her mother had been strained for many years. Her mother who had been raised in a conservative New England Protestant family was openly critical of her daughter's lifestyle. She was very upset when Susan announced that she had become pregnant and would raise the baby as a single parent. Although Mrs. Stapleton has a genuine love for her grandson, Todd, she sees him infrequently. Mr. Stapleton is even less accepting; his obstinate personality and ultra-conservative attitudes combine to interpret his approach to Susan. He treats her as if she does not exist.

As he became aware of the crisis in the Stapleton family, Reverend McEttrick, rector of the family's parish church, visited the Stapletons at their home. The pastor wished to offer his support to the family, to provide a forum in which they could express their fears and concerns, and to assist Susan in whatever ways he might.

The pastor had difficulty in getting the parents to acknowledge that Susan had been diagnosed with AIDS. Knowing her long-term involvement with drugs, he was aware of the probable diagnosis. However, Anne Stapleton was insistent that Susan had "anemia and a bad case of pneumonia, but she'll be all right." Mr. Stapleton maintained a disengaged silence throughout the pastoral visit. Reverend McEttrick met resistance with every strategy he used. Mrs. Stapleton expressed gratitude that the pastor was willing to visit Susan, but she thought that Susan would not be open to such a visit "for the time being." "Susan isn't ready to talk with anyone yet, Reverend," she said. "She's weak, and doesn't want to see many visitors; some days she isn't ready to talk to us (her parents)."

The pastor chose not to confront the Stapletons' denial, but left the door open for future work with them. "With your permission, I would be willing to call upon you at some later time if I or the parish can be of assistance to you. You can certainly call upon me at any time if either you or Susan may wish to speak with me." The pastor was prudent not to engage the family in inappropriate confrontations. He judged correctly that the family sorely needed their various expressions of denial to cope with the stressful realities of Susan's diagnosis.

Anger

In persons with AIDS, anger is a common, normal emotional response. Anger is expressed in a host of ways. The most ordinary expression is through negative verbalizations. These verbal outbursts can be strong and assaultive. Anger can be thinly masked in dark humor, sarcasm, or cynicism. It can express itself in a variety of passive-aggressive activities, non-cooperative and non-participative behaviors, and other forms of withdrawal and withholding. The basic unconscious intention behind this spectrum of negative behaviors is to punish someone who has hurt or inflicted real or imagined pain on the victim.

As with denial, anger is a normal and legitimate psychological defense. In the case of any person with AIDS, there are countless reasons which explain his or her anger. It is not necessary to chronicle these multiple sources of anger. Any person facing potential or certain death may feel anger. They see other people, comparable in age and life experience, who are well and alive. They may resent the perceived "wellness" in others, while hating the "illness" in themselves. For example, a gay man with AIDS may become angry with a lover who is not sick.

In its Scandinavian and Icelandic origins, the word "anger" means grief and sorrow. In pastoral and psychological practice, it is not uncommon to discover underneath expressions of anger an individual's more painful experiences of loss, sorrow, and grief. In order to gain access to these more important feelings, it is essential that one not react negatively to angry outbursts or attacks.

Family members and caring friends acknowledge that one of the most difficult things with which they contend in assisting a person with AIDS is dealing with expressions of anger. Anger is often targeted at those individuals who are most accessible, and, not untypically, who are the closest supports to the sick person.

Barbara Peabody recounts a family experience in *The Screaming Room*. At considerable effort and expense, Peter's sister and brothers arranged to fly to San Diego to celebrate their brother's twenty-ninth and last birthday. As it turned out, Peter slept most of the day. His mother suspected that he was more depressed than tired. "The company has been exhausting, and surely their [his siblings] energy, compared to his, is depressing."

Barbara states that the planes of her other children were scheduled to depart later that night and on the following morning. Therefore that evening would be the last opportunity for Peter to see them. They returned to the hospital to say goodbye before departing for the airport.

> *Peter is up and dressed when we return. His hair is wetly slicked down; he must have washed in the sink.*
> *"Do you want to go to the airport with us, Peter?" I ask.*
> *"No," he answers after thinking a minute. "I want to go for a walk . . . alone," he says firmly.*
> *"Can't you wait a few minutes?" I ask. "Jonathan has to leave." I am piqued by his strange rudeness.*
> *Without answering, he walks straight to David, shakes his hand, and says, "Thanks for coming. I hope you have a good trip back." Then, passing by Jonathan as if he weren't there, he rushes out the door, saying, "I have to hurry. I have to get out while there's still light." We sit, stunned, looking at one another.*
> *"Well," I say at last, "I guess that's that. Come on, let's go." I am infuriated. Was he confused, didn't know who was leaving, or what? And why so rude?*

"I don't understand that at all," I tell David and Jona-
than as we descend in the elevator. "That was really rude.
I'm sorry, Jonathan."

"Oh, that's okay, Mom. Don't worry about it. He's sick.
He doesn't always know what he's doing."

"Well, sick or not," I say indignantly, "he could at least
have walked to the car with us, as long as he was going out
anyway. He could have said goodbye. Listen, you all came
especially for his birthday, and gave up your own plans for
him. I'm really mad." I slam the car door shut. I feel hurt for
them.

"It's all right Mom," Jonathan repeats.

We leave Jonathan at his gate. There is barely time to
say goodbye.

"Let's go get some dinner, David. Tracy and Ray are
going to visit Peter tonight. He won't need extra people
around."

I'm afraid I'll explode at him if I go back. (pp. 186–187)

The next day, Barbara got up early and took David to the
airport for his return flight. Afterward, she returned to the hospital, still brooding about Peter's rude behavior to his brother.

"Good morning, Peter," I greet him when I get there.

"Where's my breakfast?" he asks in a surly tone. He's
walking back to his bed from the sink. His hyper-al(imen-
tation) tube only allows him to walk that far.

"Your breakfast?" I ask, puzzled.

"Yes, my breakfast," he repeats sarcastically. "I don't
know," I answer, bewildered. [He responds with an obscen-
ity.] "Wait a minute!" I explode. "You don't need to talk to
me that way, and I don't need to hear it. Besides, I'm tired of
you talking to me as if I were stupid. I'm not stupid and I
don't liked being talked to as if I were."

The anger, the pain, the hurt—everything is boiling up
and out of me—rage with everything, the world, AIDS, Peter,
myself. I don't even know what it is.

"I've been taking it quietly, making excuses for you—
'he's sick'—but I'm not going to take it anymore, it's just not
fair . . ." My voice starts to rise. I start to speak of his rude-

ness to his brothers, but a nurse enters and I choke back the
words.

"Think about what I said. I'll be back in a while," I tell
him as calmly as possible, storming out of the room.

I don't want to be angry with him, God knows. I know
why he's acting this way, but I can't help it. What is this
awful, pressure-cooker world we're locked in, that makes us
scream at each other when we should be loving? There's so
little time left, so little.

I push into the bathroom, dry my eyes, shove the anger
back inside, and go to the cafeteria. I cannot go back up-
stairs until I am in control of myself.

Finally, I return upstairs. Peter is quiet, docile. We
chat about insignificant matters. Any minute, a nurse will
bring a wheelchair, and we will take Peter to his new room
on the ninth floor. He will now be a human guinea pig for ten
days. [10 day experimental drug treatment with DHPG for
Cytomegalovirus] (pp. 187–188)

Caring for a person with AIDS is demanding, both physically and emotionally. The task is compounded when the person
whom you are assisting makes you the focused object of anger.
The most natural response is to retaliate, to express anger in
return. Reading Barbara Peabody's sensitive account of her relationship with her son, Peter, during his final year of struggle
with AIDS, one is aware that she tolerated a good deal of his
anger. The passages we cited from her journal illustrate a satura-
tion point in anger management.

Walking away from a person with AIDS is one strategy. It
helps to dissipate and diffuse negative feelings, provides perspective, and gives recovery time. However, it is important to interpret the walking away, since the person with AIDS may be
prone to interpret this behavior as abandonment. Perceived rejection or abandonment can intensify the aggressive and assaultive behaviors. When a person in need perceives being abandoned, he or she may experience a weakening or loss of control,
heightened anxiety, and real fears. Anger is one of the exterior
masks behind which frightened feelings play.

Pastors will encounter expressions of anger in caring for
persons with AIDS. Effective care is contingent upon a clear

understanding of the genesis of a person's anger and what it means in the context of life-threatening illness. Pastoral care may help the person better to focus anger. A pastor needs to find appropriate ways to respond to those projections of anger directed to either the Church or his or her own person. Let's review some of the more common ways in which anger is expressed.

Persons with AIDS have multiple levels of anger. Much of the anger is focused on the disease. It is appropriate that AIDS be viewed as the enemy. Many persons with AIDS direct their anger toward the virus that surreptitiously has gained access to their bodies, and silently and successfully has begun to overwhelm the body's defenses. They may be angry at those individuals whom they suspect may have been involved in transmitting the virus to them. They may be angry at medicine's inability to check the virus which is threatening their survival. Persons with AIDS may be angry at the government which may be perceived as slow to respond to the AIDS crisis. Anger may be directed at God or the Church. A person with AIDS may be angry at himself or herself for becoming infected with the virus. It is not uncommon to find many of these levels of anger in a single individual diagnosed with AIDS.

Terri is a thirty year old attractive, single, Jewish woman living in Wilmington, Delaware. After several months of diagnostic evaluations which included explorative surgery and biopsies, she was diagnosed with ARC. For the past few years she has been living with a man who is seropositive for HIV. She was unaware that he had engaged in bisexual activities. When she learned of her diagnosis, she sought the counsel of a rabbi although she did not consider herself to be religious.

The initial meetings involved helping her to manage her anger. She was enraged that her boyfriend had infected her. She was angry that as soon as her diagnosis was confirmed, he left her. Her anger was focused on her suspicion that he would infect other unsuspecting women, and that there was virtually nothing she could do to stop him, or to warn and protect other women from her fate. She was angry that her reproductive life is affected. She is angry that God allowed her to get this horrible disease.

The rabbi was comfortable with her multiple expressions of

anger. He provided her a safe haven where she could begin to give expression to the many levels of anger. He knew that her healthy adjustment to being a person with ARC was dependent upon dealing with her anger, and he was willing to assist her in this way. He was also aware that she was returning to her religious tradition seeking acceptance, understanding, support, and counsel. The rabbi's willingness and ability to become a partner with Terri in this process proved to be an effective resource for her in managing her reactions to a frightening diagnosis.

Persons with AIDS also direct their anger to the profession of medicine, to agencies of the government, toward representatives of organized religion, toward journalists and commentators in the press and electronic media. Because the AIDS pandemic is an international health problem of extraordinary scope and unprecedented urgency, it has attracted the attention and response of many sectors of society. Medicine, government, religion, and the news media each have attempted to formulate the problem and suggest appropriate responses.

Some of the ways in which the problem of AIDS is expressed by these various groups within society have infuriated persons struggling with the disease. Anger and frustration may be directed at medicine for not moving faster to discover a way to cure the disease. A person with AIDS may not be focused on the remarkable progress medicine has already made in identifying the structure of the virus and the ways in which the HIV is transmitted. Medical research continues to learn how the virus initiates infection, how it maintains infection, and what determines the progression and diversity of the illnesses associated with AIDS. However, for a person with AIDS, it seems as if medicine is impotent in the face of this disease, that doctors aren't the gods some people have thought them to be.

Anger may target the government which may be perceived as not making an adequate response to the AIDS pandemic. A person with AIDS may focus on the fact that the total amount spent on research on AIDS and HIV is a very small portion of the total funds committed to basic and applied biomedical research, development, and training. Some persons with AIDS are angry that the government, perceived as an all protective parent, has allowed this problem to reach the magnitude that it has achieved, before it became involved seriously in the fight. Some individuals may be angry at the government's proposed responses which they fear may lead to further stigmatization and quarantine.

It is never easy for a pastor to encounter anger in the context of pastoral care. Yet pastors are exposed to verbal abusiveness, aggressive and hostile accusations, sarcasm, and insult. It is difficult ministering to a person who is negative, withholding, or withdrawn. It is helpful to recall that a person with AIDS has reason to be angry, and that anger may be one strategy the person utilizes in his or her attempt to cope with an AIDS diagnosis. Anger is a common camouflage for the deeper pains of anxiety, fear, guilt, and grief. If a pastor can patiently endure the vitriol of a person's anger, he or she may be in a strategic position to assist the person to deal with the more substantive needs which the anger is masking.

3

A Light Burns in the Darkness: The Ministry of Hope to Persons with AIDS

There are many ways to describe the role of a pastor in the care of persons with AIDS. In this chapter we shall focus on an enabling role, the ministry of hope. Among people in high-risk groups where there are significant numbers of cases of AIDS, there is a perception that the whole world is dying of this disease. That perception contributes in great measure to peoples' feelings of hopelessness, depression, and despair.

Persons in the high-risk group experience double jeopardy. Not only are they members of social groups which have marginal acceptability, but now they are stigmatized further by a lethal, infectious disease. Family, friends, health care professionals, and clergy may directly or indirectly withdraw from them at a time when they are most in need. Physical and emotional distancing is experienced by persons with AIDS as abandonment and rejection. It is understandable why some individuals speak of feeling miserable, not only as a result of the effects of their illness, but because they have no one on whom they can depend. In these cases, their expressed desire to die is understandable.

While rejection is a real problem for some persons with AIDS, fortunately it is not the most common experience. The responses of family members, significant friends, health care workers, and clergy have been edifying. The recent book by Shelp, Sunderland, and Mansell, *AIDS: Personal Stories in Pas-*

39

toral Perspective (1986), chronicles many disturbing and many consoling case histories of persons with AIDS. These stories highlight the heroic efforts of people to provide love and support during the course of an individual's battle with AIDS.

Effective and consistent support helps maintain hope. We know that persons with AIDS resist being labeled as *victim*. In ancient religious usage, the term *victim* referred to a living creature that was sacrificed. In practice, a victim was a disposable commodity. During the period of the holocaust in World War II, the thousands of Jewish people sent to their death in German concentration camps were described as *victims* of the Nazis. As victims, they were expendable.

By definition, a victim has little hope. Victim implies passivity. Persons with AIDS, by rejecting the label *victim,* assert their prerogative to be treated as persons. They retain full possession of their human rights and dignity, and maintain control over their lives as long as they are alive.

The human psyche is complex. How a person thinks significantly affects how he or she feels. If a person believes that life is controllable, then he or she will work to exercise control. From research with both animal and human subjects, psychologists have concluded that there is a demonstrable relationship between psychological surrender and physical death. If the judgment is made that there is no basis for hope of living a dignified life, then a person surrenders the will to live. That decision may act as a trigger that accelerates the dying process. The following case of a thirty-two year old banker illustrates how a young man's loss of hope accelerated his death.

Graduating from an ivy league college in the northeastern United States, Jon earned a master's degree in financial management and joined a large New York banking firm. In the course of seven years with the firm he was promoted to the position of vice president in the loan department.

Early in 1986, he developed lymphadenopathy which was soon followed by a diagnosis of Pneumocystis carinii pneumonia which required his hospitalization. Jon was living with Ken who was a recent law school graduate and worked as a staff attorney in a Manhattan law firm. Jon and Ken had been in a relationship for eight months at the time of Jon's diagnosis with AIDS.

Jon was extremely depressed by his diagnosis. His sexual history could hardly be described as "fast-lane." He had been sexually active for three years prior to meeting Ken. During those years his involvements were moderate and highly selective. After meeting Ken, he had been monogamous. Although he knew a number of people who had become sick, he was certain that he wouldn't get AIDS, because he judged his own lifestyle to be safe.

He had a serious reaction to the drug he was given to treat the PCP, and his hospitalization was extended. Ken, though initially quite supportive, was finding Jon's illness to be very stressful. Balancing the excessive demands placed on a junior colleague in a high-powered law firm with primary responsibility for Jon's physical and emotional care, Ken was torn. He reasoned that if he gave Jon the kinds of support he required, his law career would be compromised. He gradually began to disengage from Jon, and soon after told him that he couldn't handle the tensions. When Jon was well enough to return to work on a reduced schedule, Ken terminated the relationship and moved out.

Jon found Ken's decision difficult, although intellectually he understood the way his former lover felt. Within three months, Jon developed a recurrent lung infection and was hospitalized again. His family lived in Cincinnati, Ohio. His parents insisted that he return to Cincinnati where they could assist in his care. Jon was not anxious to do this, although he recognized that he had few other viable options.

Jon never returned to Cincinnati; he died in the hospital in August of 1986. Those who were involved in his care described him as losing the will to live. His estrangement from Ken had a significant negative impact on him. When Ken moved out, Jon lost hope. He could see no reason to continue fighting. He did not see any future for himself. His inability to hope was nothing more than his decision to die. After Ken's departure, Jon was negligent in taking his medication and in monitoring his dietary and rest requirements. He resisted the initiatives of other friends, and chose to remain isolated. His quick relapse was not unexpected.

Let us reflect on this case. While hospitalized, Jon was depressed and did not respond to overtures made to him by social services or pastoral care. Therefore, the analysis of this case is speculative. What did AIDS mean to Jon? For him it signaled a significant interruption of his promising career. It placed major burdens on the interpersonal relationship he was developing with Ken, to such a degree that the relationship was destroyed. AIDS necessitated disclosure to his parents about his homosexuality. Although they were upset by the dual disclosure, they were accepting and wanted him to come home. But the prospect of having to become dependent upon them for future care was something he was reluctant to accept.

Each of these personal meanings contributed to his feelings of hopelessness. His behavioral responses were consistent with this pervasive hopelessness. He was not vigilant in maintaining his general health by proper rest and diet. He became socially withdrawn, even reclusive. Gradually he surrendered the will to live. Having relapsed within three months, he had little motivation to fight, and he succumbed more quickly than other persons with a similar history of infections.

Two issues of general significance to helping persons with AIDS to maintain hope are worthy of mention. The first is the issue of support. It is difficult to sustain hope in the face of uncertainty unless there is real and perceived support. Ken's departure was not only a real loss of support, but it became symbolic as well. There may be many sources of support available; some people appear unable to use these resources. Jon was in this latter group. He refused offers of support from parents, colleagues and friends, and from the professionals involved in his care, including pastoral care. Without effective support, his hopes for life evaporated quickly.

A second issue has to do with control. Jon's diagnosis of AIDS upset the delicate balance of controls in his life. His career began to race out of control, his relationship was short-circuited, his ability to make prudent decisions about health maintenance was lost. His future appeared bleak and his options narrowed. He rejected the offer to return home, and to, in effect, surrender control for his life to his parents who offered to care for him.

Jon's case raises some important questions about the proper role of family and professional intervention with persons who appear to surrender the will to live. For the purposes of this discussion, we shall restrict our focus to the appropriateness of pastoral intervention. Should a pastor have attempted to break through Jon's resistance? Should a pastor have worked to help Jon accept support and try to regain control over his life? In his book *Love, Medicine, and Miracles* (1986), Bernard S. Siegel reflects on his extensive work in self-healing with exceptional cancer patients. In this professional engagement, Dr. Siegel continually confronts the value question of continued life. "It's not for us to evaluate the worth of continued life for another person," states Siegel. "As long as my patients are living in a way that has value for them, I'm there to help them continue." A pastor might benefit from reflection on this philosophical principle of care.

Pastors must diligently avoid projecting their own values of continued life onto a person with AIDS. One can communicate verbal and non-verbal messages of support and understanding. However, for some individuals, AIDS means death, and they may find little meaning in attempting to live with AIDS. For others—and experience supports the judgment that this represents the majority of persons with AIDS—AIDS presents a formidable challenge to live, despite the present lack of a definitive medical cure for this life-threatening disease. It is to this population of persons who choose to live with AIDS that we now turn our attention. To borrow Siegel's expression, we want to understand better how persons with AIDS "are living in a way that has value for them," and how as pastors we can "help them continue."

How Are Persons with AIDS Living?

In *The Screaming Room,* from which we have already excerpted, Barbara Peabody recalls her son Peter's early determination to live. In her entry dated Monday, 2 January, she recalls a conversation with Peter after he had made telephone contact with another person with AIDS who was a volunteer at the Gay Men's Health Crisis in New York City.

> *He was so encouraging, so positive. He started out by asking how I felt about a lot of things, and I told him I was a little worried about what might happen. So he asked me, "Do you want to live?" and I said, "Of course," and he said, "Then*

you will, you'll find a way." It was really good to talk to him
(p. 41).

Peter's mother was riveted on what Bob Cecci had told her son, and what Peter's reactions were. She asked Peter whether Bob shared how he was coping with AIDS. Peter answered affirmatively and shared the following:

> *He says it has been getting to him lately—there've been several deaths—and he's been told he should take a week or two off and rest. But he said that he feels AIDS has been a positive force for him, made him stop and think exactly what he wants, which he never bothered to do before. He says it forced him to re-evaluate his life, and how he feels he has something special to contribute and something to live for. I told him that's the way I've been feeling, too, and that I want to do some volunteer work in California. He said he thought I'd do fine and wished me luck. He's such a sincere person . . . (p. 42).*

Barbara concludes her entry for that date with the following words: "I'm delighted with Peter's excited eagerness to live, to make something good out of something so evil and negative. I hope this will keep up a long, long time."

There are many variables that contribute to the determination of a person with AIDS to live. It will be helpful to identify and comment upon some of these resources.

Principal Relationships

Barbara Peabody's story documenting the love and dedication that sustained her relationship with her son Peter during his struggle with AIDS is a useful starting point. Her story is repeated in the life of every person with AIDS who has been able to sustain hope in the face of this disease. Whether it is a parent, sibling, lover, friend, or priest, a person with AIDS needs a deeper relationship with someone. The needs in terms of physical care are evident, and should not been minimized in any discussion. However, the emotional and spiritual dimensions of a deeper interpersonal relationship deserve further exploration.

The decision to attempt to live with AIDS exposes some of the most profound human feelings. They run the spectrum from moments of exhilaration to moments of despair; from great optimism about a new treatment or drug, to profound disappointment when it does not prove to be the hoped-for remedy. There are moments of almost symbiotic closeness and times of frightening distance, of tenderness and warmth, of hardness and stoic disregard. These are but some of the multiple and changing faces of relationship with a person with AIDS. Constancy binds together the fabric of these transformations. The sense that "we'll see this through together" forms the *cantus firmus* of all successful relationships with persons with AIDS.

Marianne and Glen Redding met Father Toland when Glen was hospitalized and diagnosed with AIDS in March of 1984. A lifelong hemophiliac, Glen depended on many transfusions of blood products containing the clotting agent, Factor VIII.

Hemophilia is a genetically inherited clotting disorder. The blood of a hemophiliac lacks Factor VIII, and thus the person is vulnerable to prolonged and life-threatening bleeding, even from something as ordinary as a minor cut. To prepare the Factor VIII blood product, the plasma from 2,500 to 10,000 donors may be utilized. It is probable that Glen contracted AIDS through this route of transmission.

Father Toland was a parish priest in the community in which Marianne and Glen resided. At the time of Glen's diagnosis, they were not actively practicing Catholics, although both had been raised in that religious tradition. The Reddings had been married for three years when Glen was diagnosed. Marianne was three months pregnant with their first child. Over the course of the next twenty-two months prior to Glen's death, Father Toland became a close friend to the Reddings, spending time regularly with them in their home and during Glen's subsequent four hospitalizations.

Marianne recalls the immediate rapport Father Toland was able to establish with them, and the highlights of the relationship he maintained throughout Glen's illness.

He was gentle and caring. Neither of us ever felt that he was burdened by the time he spent with us. He seemed to

*understand what we were feeling before we could even ex-
press it. And the times when we couldn't express it, we were
sure he knew.*

*When Todd was born in September 1984, Glen was in
the hospital again. Father Toland was there for both of us;
he was like an expectant father, awaiting the results of my
delivery (the baby seems OK, thank God!). His excitement
was infectious. Glen said that Father Toland seemed more
excited by Todd's birth than even he felt. Of course, Glen was
very excited. I think it helped him to keep fighting so that he
could enjoy sharing our firstborn's life together.*

*Over the last couple of years, Father Toland has become
the most important person in our lives. There were many
times that we forgot he was a priest. He was just our best
friend, even closer than our families who have been tremendously supportive throughout the long ordeal. He was special. He was constantly calling, offering to run to the store,
babysit Todd, cook a meal, drive Glen to see his doctor, take
us for a ride to see the autumn foliage. In all of this, he
helped us to rediscover our relationship to God, not by
preaching, but by the countless, wonderful ways in which he
was always there for us. Although we both have tried to
express what he has meant to us, and continues to mean to
me, I don't think we could adequately express this. Too bad
there aren't more priests like Father Toland in the Catholic
Church . . .*

"I don't know why he ever took an interest in a druggie like
me," was the way Beth began to relate the story of her relationship with Paul Roche. Paul was a third-year divinity student,
preparing for ordination in the Episcopal Church. He was involved in a clinical pastoral internship program in a large university hospital where Beth was admitted with PCP. She was a
twenty-eight year old woman who had left home when she was
seventeen years old. During the intervening years she had been
heavily involved in abuse of a variety of drugs, including the
intravenous injection of heroin. Her weight loss, anemia, and
pneumonia substantiated her AIDS diagnosis.

Estranged from her family who were from a conservative

Protestant tradition, Beth was reluctant to reestablish contact with them. "They consider me dead, already," she said. "They want to forget they ever had a daughter who turned out to be a dope addict and who now has AIDS." Beth's characterization of her parents sadly proved to be correct.

With her reluctant permission, her doctor contacted her parents. Her father received the information about Beth's condition with cold indifference, saying that he and his wife could not become involved with their daughter whom they had not seen in more than eight years. What he clearly communicated, though he did not directly verbalize his judgment, was that Beth brought this situation on herself and that she would have to live with the consequences of her behavior. It was clear that he was unwilling to provide any assistance in her care. When her physician communicated the fact that he had made contact with her father, she said: "Well, now you know what I told you."

Beth was hesitant to trust the relationship that Paul Roche attempted to build with her during her seven-week hospitalization. Initially, she was assigned to him as a pastoral care patient. This was Paul's first encounter with a person with AIDS. Hardened by her street experiences, Beth was instinctively distrustful. Paul did not force the relationship, but found time each day to sit with her. Beth commented that she never found Paul "blaming me for my past." He was successful in communicating acceptance, empathy, and genuine concern. He spoke to her about her future, was helpful in talking to the hospital's Department of Social Services about discharge plans, and was invested in trying to keep her hopes alive.

Paul experienced great conflicts as he faced the necessity of termination. At the conclusion of his internship he would be returning to his seminary in another state. With the help of his supervisor, he began to work through the delicate issues of withdrawing from a patient who had grown attached to him. Beth was dependent on his presence and support. Paul was able to introduce another permanent chaplain to Beth and gradually to transfer responsibilities for her pastoral care to him.

What Paul was able to accomplish during his brief but intensive pastoral relationship with Beth helped her to explore and diffuse her guilt for the abusive life she had led which contrib-

uted to her AIDS diagnosis. His hopeful and constructive interventions helped her to maintain a will to live, despite familial
abandonment. The case points out what a short-term relationship can do to facilitate a person's desire to live, even when there
may be no ostensible reason to do so.

Ted and Andy met the summer after they graduated from
college. In their words it was "love at first sight." They shared a
very simple apartment on 89th Street in New York City. Ted was
a drama and voice major in college, and was attempting to break
into the competitive New York theater, while working as a
waiter until he got his big break. Andy had accepted a promising
job as a graphic artist with an advertising firm. Their life together during the first two years of their relationship was reward-
ing, and their commitment to each other was deepening.

In August of 1986 Andy first noticed some pink spots on
Ted's chest. At first they were not terribly visible, because Ted's
chest was very hairy, and the lesions were camouflaged. Andy
felt the bumps, and suspected they were acne pimples. Ted
disregarded them entirely. They persisted, darkened, and became more hard to the touch. Andy insisted that Ted have them
checked, fearing that they could be Kaposi's sarcoma lesions,
but Andy was afraid to even verbalize his fear.

With his continued pressure, Andy finally persuaded Ted
to be checked, and accompanied him to the outpatient clinic
at Saint Vincent's Hospital in Greenwich Village. After a biopsy was done and the results reviewed, the diagnosis of Kaposi's sarcoma was confirmed. Ted was treated on an outpatient basis.

Andy became very involved in helping Ted make some radical lifestyle changes. They stopped going out to the bars; there
were no more all night parties. Andy got a number of books on
nutrition, and together they began to alter their diet. They became involved in a regular program of exercise.

Ted is highly motivated to remain as healthy as possible. In
his case, the lesions have not spread, and he has not had any
other serious opportunistic infections during the past year. In
reflecting on Andy's role in his attitudes towards AIDS, Ted said
the following:

*I don't know what I would have done if Andy and I did
not have the relationship we do. I haven't told my family
about it (AIDS), and I hope I never have to. It would kill
them to find out. Andy has helped me to think that I might be
able to beat this if I do everything possible to remain healthy.
Not only has he turned my life around during the past year,
but he has also done a lot to change the way I think about
life. He is the best friend I have in the world. I have a feeling
he will always be there for me.*

In each of these case vignettes, the importance of a deep
human relationship for maintaining a commitment to live is
evident. In some of these cases, the relationship involves primary responsibilities for providing physical care. In other cases,
those responsibilities may be discharged by a number of persons, while the principal emotional needs of the person with
AIDS are addressed by one individual.

Pastors frequently find themselves in the latter category. In
the case of Father Toland, who became involved in some additional supportive activities with the Redding family during the
course of Glen's terminal struggle with AIDS, a pastor may find
himself or herself moving out of traditional ministerial roles.
Pastoral care attempts to enkindle and sustain hope in the face
of the serious challenges which AIDS presents. The ability of
the pastor to forge a deeper relationship with the individual with
AIDS and his or her family can influence significantly not only
the effectiveness of spiritual ministrations, but the person's very
will to live.

Changing One's Mental Outlook

For centuries people have struggled to answer the question
of the intrinsic relationship between mind and body. The question has been formulated differently. While academicians continue to debate the issue, few dispute the essential relationship
that exists between mind and body.

Persons involved in the practice of dynamic psychotherapy
know experientially that if one is successful in helping persons

alter the ways in which they think about themselves or about a particularly distressing issue, a change in thinking will affect both bodily functions and behavior.

Pastoral care implicitly has been engaged in helping people change the ways in which they think about many aspects of their lives. In the Judaeo-Christian tradition, the Scriptures have been read and explained to help people modify the ways in which they understand and live their relationship to God and to each other. The work of conversion involves the work of changing one's thinking in order to change one's behavior. The work of reconciliation includes helping a person to see what is disordered in his or her approach to life and relationships, and to commit oneself to act upon what one sees. The traditional religious notion of inspiration appeals to a divine influence directly and immediately exerted on the mind or heart of a person. The significance of such inspiration is apparent: a person is animated, influenced, affected to such a degree that the body actively responds and behavior is changed.

The consoling ministries of the Church strive to help people discover inner peacefulness. Peacefulness is more than a static state of harmony, serenity, or tranquility. Achieving peace of mind involves active engagement in the tasks of confronting and challenging the mental outlooks that threaten the very foundations of bodily health.

If the work of pastoral care is successful, a person will be involved in changing those mental outlooks that compromise bodily health and integrity. From a holistic perspective, the relationship between effective pastoral care and physical health is assumed. Let us look at some of the ways in which pastoral care to persons with AIDS can influence bodily health.

Pastor Schmidt provided volunteer support to an inpatient hospice program in the local community hospital. Kristin was a thirty-one year old woman who had been involved in both drugs and prostitution, and was diagnosed with Pneumocystis carinii pneumonia and Cytomegalovirus. She was hospitalized in a community hospital for several weeks, and her condition was deteriorating. She was minimally responsive to the various drugs that were employed to treat her multiple infections.

Kristin was moved to the hospice wing of the hospital at her request. She also asked to see a Lutheran pastor since she had been raised in a very strict Lutheran family in rural Wisconsin. Although she was very weak, she was anxious to talk with Pastor Schmidt. Quickly she told him her story, outlining her long involvement in drugs and prostitution. He was able to listen to her self-disclosures with attention and compassion.

In ministering to her, he chose to read and discuss the graphic story of the adulteress in Chapter 8 of the Gospel of John. The story chronicles the quick-moving events of a woman's adultery, discovery, apprehension by Jewish officials, and their resolve to stone her to death, a punishment directed by the strict interpretation of the law. Asking Jesus for his interpretation of their duty, Jesus replied: "Let the person who is without sin among you be the first to cast a stone at her." One by one they departed, until the woman stood alone with Jesus. "Has no one condemned you?" "No one, Lord," she replied. "Neither will I condemn you. Go your way and reform your life."

Kristin's eyes began to tear as the pastor read these words and began to apply them in analogous ways to her own personal life. He spoke in a gentle and loving way about God's compassion and willingness to forgive. His manner of relating to Kristin was respectful and his words were inspiring, avoiding any sense that she was to blame for her present illness. He spoke to her about hope, saying that she should not allow this illness to "stone" her.

Pastor Schmidt continued to visit her. Her physical condition began to show some modest signs of improvement, but her mental attitudes began to change more dramatically. The nurses noted what one of them termed a "reengagement with life." Kristin told one of them, "If my former lifestyle played some role in my getting AIDS, then I can use whatever energies I have left to begin to turn things around." Pastor Schmidt's work with her, focused on forgiveness, self-acceptance, and hope, played a central role in her attitude change, and her new determination to live.

Kristin died in the hospice thirteen weeks after her admission. During the final weeks of her life she achieved reconciliation with some members of her family through telephone conversations. One of her brothers flew east to be with her and assumed responsibility for bringing her body back to Wisconsin for burial. Kristin died peacefully. Her final weeks of life were important in helping her to affirm her personal worth. In an ironic sense, her terminal diagnosis with AIDS helped her discover a deeper meaning to her life.

Few persons with AIDS want to think about the disease as a *terminal* illness. In Barbara Peabody's journal, *The Screaming Room*, Peter raised the question: "Well, what do you think is a good word for AIDS?" The following is the entry for 13 September:

> *"Let's see . . ." I answer, thinking. The word* terminal *is very offensive to Peter, as is the word* victim, *instead of* patient *to many others. "It is a chronic disease, but it's more serious than that. I've seen it referred to as life-threatening. That implies the inherent danger but not the absolute finality of terminal."*
>
> *"Yes . . . yes, I think life-threatening is good," Peter agrees.*
>
> *(Speaking to his nurse, Phyllis, Peter says:) " . . . After all, you can't call a disease terminal when only 45 percent of the cases have died, not 100 percent. Some have lived three to five years, and records have only been kept since 1981. How do you know that they're all going to die? I think that terminal is insulting, offensive to the patient, because it takes away all his hope and can discourage him immediately. And hope is a very important part of the patient's mental and physical health, and essential if he's going to get any better and not give in. It's not fair to take away someone's chances for survival by taking away his hope, and if he's told that he has a terminal disease, that's just what you do, right at the start"—he pauses a minute, tired from such a long speech.*
>
> *"You have a good point, Peter," Phyllis agrees pensively.*
>
> *"It just makes me angry to hear people call AIDS terminal, that's all," he tells her.*
>
> *"I really appreciate your talking to me about it," Phyllis says. "The medical community often gets so wrapped up in its professional and technical approach to disease that it forgets about the patient's feelings, and that those feelings are very important to his well-being. I'm glad you told me this, because we need to know what the patient feels. We can*

empathize only so far. The patient ultimately is the only one who knows how he feels" (pp. 191–92).

Peter's conversation on the significance of the adjective *terminal* to describe AIDS, stimulated Barbara Peabody's own reflections. She concludes her entry with these words:

> *I do think Peter has a valid point, and he has become an expert on survival, after all. His physical resources would have been hopelessly inadequate without the emotional impetus his hope has given him.*
>
> *His indomitable will to survive continues to amaze me. Despite all his talents and intelligence, Peter has never been able to set goals for himself and fulfill them. He's always been too easily discouraged and let plans fall apart at the slightest setback or disappointment. And now, here he is, barely surviving—but indeed surviving. It's as if he's made survival the purpose of his life, to prove to himself and others that this strange and vicious disease can indeed be battled, and that Peter Vom Lehn is going to win. It is his greatest challenge and he has met it head-on and unflinching. I don't think he has any long-term goals such as what he would do with his life if he should be cured. Maybe he'd find himself with nothing to do. But at this point, it hardly matters (pp. 192–193).*

Peter's concerns about the use of the word *terminal* to describe AIDS highlight the importance of language in coloring how a person thinks about a disease. In order to maintain hope and engagement with life, a person needs to think there is some possibility of survival. The struggle to survive, as Peter's case so poignantly demonstrates, is formidable. His determination to beat the odds is bolstered by his acknowledgement that while AIDS is *life-threatening,* there is the possibility of control while hoping for the discovery of a cure.

As pastors, we need to be sensitive to the ways in which we talk about disease. Just as nurses can use words like *lethal* and *terminal* while providing ordinary care to persons with AIDS, a pastor can inadvertently use the same language. Unconsciously, language can destroy a person's hope, take away the challenge to survive, and force an individual to surrender the remaining controls he or she has over life. To recall the premise stated earlier, how persons think affects how they feel. If they think of themselves as terminally ill, they will begin to prepare for death. On the other hand, if they think of themselves as confronted with a life-threatening illness, they will be more prepared to attempt to survive the threat.

Some Practical Ways To Support a Person's Hopes

In the practice of pastoral care with persons with AIDS, there are some specific ways to assist a person maintain a positive and engaged approach to life. Too often pastors feel impotent in the face of the overwhelming needs and problems they encounter in persons with AIDS. In subsequent chapters we will consider the needs of care-providers and families. Now we shall focus our attention on the care of persons with AIDS.

Assess the Person's Philosophy of Life

It is imperative that the pastor understand what the person with AIDS holds as life's values. It may take some time to create the appropriate emotional climate in which a person is willing to share these important values. Not only is it important to understand these personal values, but the pastor needs to communicate acceptance of these values. Acceptance does not imply agreement. Some pastors find it difficult to make this distinction. In working with persons with AIDS, it is to be anticipated that some of the expressed values of persons in the high-risk groups afflicted by this disease will not be endorsed by some religious faiths. Just as counselors must learn to be non-judgmental in dealing with clients' values at odds with their own, so too must pastors appropriate these attitudes in their work with persons with AIDS.

Express Empathy

A person with AIDS needs to feel that a prospective helper understands his or her inner struggles. While intellectual understanding is an indispensable starting point, the person with AIDS is helped when the pastor is effective in communicating that he or she also understands and shares the individual's feelings. In speaking of her relationship with her pastor, a twenty-six year old mother with ARC whose two year old son was diagnosed with AIDS said:

> *Reverend Cantwell is a very caring woman. She has become such a good friend to me, even though I have hardly been what you would call a "church-going person." She listens to everything I say, and makes me feel good about myself. At times I feel real guilty about giving my son AIDS, wondering if he'll hate his mom for this, but Rev. Cantwell is right there to help me. She's a mother, and I think she feels what I'm feeling. That makes me feel so much better. There are many times I forget she's a Reverend, and I think of her more as my older sister.*

Maintain a Positive Outlook

In speaking about AIDS, there is a problem in finding anything positive to say. In working with persons with AIDS, there is a similar danger that the orientation in conversation may be negatively skewed. In order to maintain a person's realistic hopes in the face of this disease, efforts must be focused on reinforcing positive gains. This might involve helping a person to communicate directly with parents or friends. It could involve resuming work on a limited schedule. Gaining two pounds might be an important milestone, or having a day without a debilitating reaction to a therapeutic drug.

Pastors should be alert to identify and respond to these cues. Person's with AIDS need to find encouragement in efforts they may be making to survive. They need others to recognize the small gains they may be achieving.

In February, 1986, Leo was diagnosed with Kaposi's sarcoma. Since his diagnosis, the lesions have not appeared in other places on his body, and he has not had any other opportunistic infections. He is actively involved in a local chapter of Persons With AIDS. During a recent clinic visit, his doctor was commenting on the very positive attitude Leo displayed, and his evident lifestyle changes. Leo attributed much of the changes to his support system. He made particular reference to his relationship with Fr. Brayley whom he met through the Dignity [a support group for gay Catholics] chapter to which he belongs.

Since my crisis last February, Fr. Bob (Brayley) has been a very important person in my life. I became active again in the Church after I was diagnosed. Maybe I was afraid I would die, and turned back to God. It was fortunate I did. Fr. Bob has helped me get my life back on track. He has made me feel real positive about the things I've been doing. He has never let me forget how important I am, first to myself and to others.

I found myself asking: "What would Fr. Bob think about this or that?" I know he is in my corner, cheering me on. The fact that I've been as healthy as I think I've been these past few months is due to the things I've been doing to eat better, to get more rest, to get my head straight. And everything I succeed in doing, Fr. Bob is there to support me and encourage me. And he has even got me back praying and going to Mass. That, in itself, is no small miracle . . .

Support Independent Decision-Making and Activities

It is easy to think of all persons with AIDS as handicapped, requiring special assistance. At some stages of the illness and when the disease expresses itself in certain ways, a person may need particular forms of physical support. In general, it is important to help the person with AIDS to maintain autonomy, to retain control of his or her decisions and behaviors.

It is not uncommon to note among the behaviors of sick persons a certain amount of regression. This is evident in their passivity, their abrogation of decision-making, their expectations that others should take care of all their basic needs. These are normal reactions to illness, and the behaviors are sanctioned by our social mores. However, if these regressive tendencies are not challenged appropriately, a person can lose the motivation to recover. Some people adopt the "sick role" as a habitual mode of being, and resist getting better.

Some of these psychological dynamics, common to many

individuals with acute illnesses, are observable in some people with AIDS. Care-providers must be able to strike a balance between providing necessary services and creating a situation of over-dependency.

In pastoral care, the pastor needs to be aware of the potentially counterproductive effects of an overly paternalistic approach. Paternalism is expressed not only in behaviors, but also in language. While paternal words and gestures might appear to be accepted by the sick individual and be comforting, at the same time they can contribute to passivity and dependence. Pastoral care should strive to create an environment where the individual feels encouraged to do more for himself or herself, knowing that he or she has support. Interventions should aim to help the person seek personal solutions to problems, rather than solving problems for the person. Depression results when others take control and solve problems. A person needs to determine goals and decide ways to achieve those goals.

An effective model of this strategy of pastoral care is found in the Christian Gospel in Luke 5:18–26. In that passage, a group of men carried a paralyzed man on a pallet and placed him before Jesus, hoping that he would cure him. In this situation, the paralyzed person needed physical assistance. This was an appropriate use of other people's assistance.

There were enormous crowds in Capernaum around the house in which Jesus was staying, so they had to climb up and lower the man through the roof. Recognizing their determination and faith, Jesus expressed forgiveness and healed the man. His dismissal to the formerly paralyzed man was: "Arise, take up your bed and go home." And the evangelist records that the man immediately arose, took up what he had been lying on, and went away to his house, glorifying God.

Jesus placed direct responsibility for the future on the formerly paralyzed individual. He didn't say to the others, "Take his bed home for him." Healing is linked with belief and personal action. Pastoral care should attempt to facilitate both.

Pastoral care of persons with AIDS should be enabling, encouraging, supportive. It should foster independence of thinking and choosing. It should create a feeling of partnership, rather than of paternalism.

Our Savior's Episcopal Church was host for a weekly nondenominational support group for persons with AIDS and ARC. The group was formed and facilitated by Rev. Clayton Reynolds, rector of Our Savior's. Since its formation in 1985, the group has provided a helping forum for dozens of persons with AIDS and ARC. Reynolds, aged sixty-one, co-leads the group with his assistant, Rev. Stephanie Chase, whose son died of AIDS in August of 1983. Mrs. Chase was ordained an Episcopal priest in 1985 and was assigned to Our Savior's. She was already involved in AIDS ministry, and was instrumental, along with Rev. Reynolds, in founding the support group.

Both priests have an open and caring attitude toward the people who participate in this group. Reynolds' and Chase's styles of participation as leaders are different. Reynolds tends to be more measured in what he says, speaking infrequently in group discussions. Chase, on the other hand, is more animated, responsive, often intervening to summarize or clarify feelings. Both of them support the "Take up your bed and walk" approach to pastoral care. And this philosophy of AIDS ministry appears to be effective.

The group traditionally ends with a brief prayer service. The thrust of the prayers, led by either of the two group facilitators, is always enabling and hopeful. In essence, they ask God continually to help these people find better ways to help themselves.

Foster Integrity, Self-Acceptance, and Love

In his classic book, *On Dying and Denying: A Psychiatric Study of Terminality* (1972), Avery Weisman talked about hope as it relates to perceived self-worth and self-acceptance.

> Hope, however, is not dependent upon survival alone. . . . Hope means that we have confidence in the *desirability* of survival. It arises from a desirable self-image, healthy self-esteem, and belief in our ability to exert a degree of influence on the world surrounding us. . . .

> Hope is decided more by self-acceptance than by objects sought and by impractical aspirations. . . . Foreshortened life does not in itself create hopelessness. . . . More im-

portant is our belief that we do something worth doing, and that others think so, too. Thus, people lose hope when they are unable to act on their own behalf and must also relinquish their claims upon others (pp. 20–21).

Speaking in the same vein in *Love, Medicine, and Miracles* (1986), Bernie Siegel notes: "Hoping means seeing that the outcome you want is possible, and then working for it" (p. 178). The purpose of any form of assistance to persons with AIDS should be to help the individual to achieve personal goals. Integrity, self-acceptance, and love are necessary, common, and realizable goals.

Integrity, self-acceptance, and love imply emotional honesty. For some individuals, AIDS exposes areas of one's personal life that have been hidden or inadequately addressed. When psychologists talk about self-acceptance, they are referring to open engagement with the ideas, perceptions, assumptions, and beliefs that a person has about himself. Although many of us have certain self-focused beliefs, we may not be fully aware of all the beliefs we hold about ourselves.

Life-threatening illness can expose hidden aspects of the self. Effective pastoral care can help an individual to explore, accept, and integrate these various aspects of the self. How a person perceives himself or herself will act as a powerful determinant in how he or she acts.

At the time of his diagnosis with Pneumocystis carinii pneumonia, Mike was two weeks short of his twenty-third birthday. Since he was sixteen years old he had been living on his own. His parents were divorced when he was eight years old, and until his departure from home he had been living with his mother and her various boyfriends. He worked in a number of minimum wage jobs and lived with two roommates in a rundown section of the city. To support his drug dependency, Mike also had been involved in male prostitution in Boston.

Admitted to a municipal hospital, he was visited by a staff chaplain who was able to establish rapport with him. This was fortuitous, since few others on the staff had been able to break through to him. Mike had not been raised in any religious tradition, although his parents had both been nominal Catholics.

Mike seemed intrigued by the accent of Fr. Sean O'Flaherty, a native of Ireland, who was working at the hospital as part of his internship experience in pastoral counseling. O'Flaherty was a doctoral candidate in the Psychology of Religion and Pastoral Counseling program at Boston University.

Mike was angry and depressed. He had few visitors. His roommates were frightened by his diagnosis of AIDS and told him that he couldn't return to the apartment but would have to find someplace else to live. Mike suspected he got AIDS from one of his male customers, although it would be difficult to determine if this were so. He had shared needles with others in intravenous drug use.

O'Flaherty visited him almost daily during the five weeks in which he was hospitalized. Gradually Mike was willing to open up to the priest, telling him his life story. He was able to ventilate his frustrations, anger, doubts, and fears. Alienated from his mother whom he had not seen in more than five years, discouraged, and depressed, Mike openly spoke of suicide as a "way to end it all." "If I'm going to die of AIDS, I might as well do it now." O'Flaherty listened more than he talked. It was clear to him that Mike had few reasons to live.

The nineteenth century German philosopher, Friedrich Nietzsche, emphasized the importance of the *will to power* as the chief motivating force of both individual and society. He asserted that the person who has the *why* to live can endure almost any *how*. Finding the reason to live is the key to survival.

In his conversations with Mike, Fr. O'Flaherty tried to help his young friend to recognize and affirm his basic worth. He was able to help him to accept that he was liked, that he was cared for, that there were some people who wanted to help him. With the help of a local AIDS Action Committee, O'Flaherty was able to make some initial arrangements for housing and assistance after he was discharged. Mike's attitudes toward his illness began to change and he began to express some realistic, short-range goals.

They never talked specifically about religion, although all of what O'Flaherty was able to do with this disengaged, depressed young man gave flesh to the saying of Jesus: "I came that you might have life, and know it in all of its fullness" (Jn 10:10).

In many of the pastoral care interventions cited in this chapter, we have seen how clergy have been effective in bringing some glimmer of hope to the darkness of the world of a person with AIDS. As persons with AIDS frequently acknowledge, they depend upon these caring partnerships to keep their hopes alive.

4

The Issues of Sexuality and Death
In AIDS Pastoral Care

To become involved in the pastoral care of persons with AIDS, a pastor confronts basic human experiences of sexuality and death. These are issues which trigger feelings of anxiety and discomfort in many people. Social and religious traditions have sanctioned avoidance of these topics in public discussion. AIDS has demanded that society face directly these two issues and dialogue with them. Both society and the Church reluctantly entertain this discussion, emotionally unprepared for the engagement.

It is not the purpose of this chapter to debate further the traditional attitudes of Western society and Judaeo-Christian religions toward sexuality and death. Rather, the purpose of this discussion will be to highlight how these two issues affect ministry to persons with AIDS. Each pastor is encouraged to reflect upon his or her thoughts, attitudes, and feelings, and to formulate anew his or her position on sexuality and death. All of us in the helping professions are aware that our attitudes and values, conscious and unconscious, are brought to bear on the relationships we have with those whom we attempt to help. In order to be of maximum effectiveness in our pastoral care of persons with AIDS, we must have informed positions and compassionate approaches in working with these two issues.

SEXUALITY

Sexuality: Pastoral-Theological Perspectives

There have been many attempts to describe the function of sexuality in human growth and development. Developmental psychologists, regardless of theoretical orientation, support the assertion that sexuality is an integral and indispensable component of human personality. Many would go further and state that sexuality is one of the most important components of human development, the physiological and psychological foundation for the capacity to love. We are by nature social beings, and thus we are in relationship with each other. Our sexuality is the context in which we enter these relationships, through which we are able to realize our human potential.

The Western Christian tradition, on the other hand, has considered sexuality principally in terms of its reproductive function. It locates the moral exercise of human reproductive activity solely within lawful marriage. There is little or no evidence within this tradition that sexuality is understood as the affective dynamic in all significant human relating. An understanding of sexuality as affective energy is not explicitly presented in the Bible. Though the history of thought on this subject is complex, a number of factors are significant in accounting for a mainly genital understanding of human sexuality.

Marriage and the family were already long established institutions by the beginning of the Judaeo-Christian era. From the beginning marriage was considered a sacred union among Christian couples and is regarded as sacramental by many ecclesial traditions. Despite the premium placed on virginity in the early Church, children were always defended as good and were seen as adding to the human race and to the kingdom of heaven as well. While orthodox writers and preachers condemned extramarital and non-marital sexual behaviors which were sometimes linked to religious and doctrinal aberrations, they vindicated marital procreational activity.

In a parallel development, the stoic outlook of the time led many Fathers of the Church to depreciate human emotion. Augustine considered sexual pleasure even in marriage to be tainted by original sin and hence tolerable only in light of procreative purpose. Such judgments had incalculable effects on later centuries. The patristic legacy was reinforced by Church discipline and the penitential codes which judged behaviors. This discipline was negative to most sexual behaviors. These trends in the disciplines concerning the expression of sexuality convinced later generations that sexual feelings were suspect, and that sexual activity was inherently marital and procreational in nature. It was to be expected that human sexuality would be subject to control by legal and moral norms, and this helps explain the guilt that many in our tradition have associated with sexual feelings and actions. As this tradition evolved, there was no recognition of sexuality as having a primary relational importance.

It would be a mistake to conclude that the Western Christian tradition was blind to human relationships. On the contrary, the Church has viewed itself as the community of those reconciled to God in Christ, a community with the mission to witness and extend this reconciliation to all. Relationships emerge as dominant not only in marriage and family, but also in friendships and in religious orders and similar groups. However important these various communities have been, it remains true that they have not generally been examined or explained through the prism of human sexuality as affective interpersonal dynamic.

In the Scholastic era, this inheritance was dominant. Natural law argumentation of a differentiated and nuanced kind, supported this rigorous sexual ethic. In the post-Reformation period, churches reinforced a strict sexual ethic. Jansenism in Roman Catholicism and the growth of puritan and fundamentalist groups in Protestantism were examples of this trend. The tendency to strictness not infrequently has led to a pastoral practice that is rigoristic and judgmental of persons who do not measure up.

In sum, this is our legacy. Sexuality is about genital behaviors that have religious and moral significance. The inheritance has a behavioral control orientation. In this scheme, only marital and procreative intercourse is legitimated.

It is only since the turn of this century that we have discovered the cultural, philosophical, and religious framework needed to sustain a discussion of sexuality in terms of human affective relating. In the Roman Catholic Church an emerging personalistic outlook has allowed the definitive affirmation of a unitive aspect to marriage and marital intercourse. Yet this new emphasis remains limited in its application. It has not extended to human relationships generally, and does not, in official teachings, allow any displacement of the procreational and behavioral requirements still dominant in Catholic sexual ethics.

There have been few attempts to articulate a new theology of sexuality within the traditional Christian churches. If such a theology were to be expressed, it would need to draw from the Scriptures a sexually sensitive understanding of relationships, while affirming the procreational dimensions.

In such a theology sexuality would be situated within the context of God's creative plan and purpose. God not only created things, but he placed those things in a hierarchy of relationships to himself and to other persons. If we remind ourselves of the creation narratives in the opening chapters of the Hebrew Scriptures, we note the author's insistence that God was pleased with the work of his hand. "And God saw that it was good" is the constant refrain in the Genesis account. Each part of his creative act had a relationship to the whole. To observe creation in harmony was a source of gratification to the Creator.

With dramatic effect, human persons were created. "God created man in his image. In the image of God he created him, male and female he created them" (Gen 1:27). Man and woman are the final acts of creation, placed in a superior relationship to the rest of the created order. In describing the creation of man, the author of Genesis notes that "the Lord God formed man out of the dust of the ground and breathed into his nostrils the breath of life, and man became a living being" (Gen 2:7).

The ancient, primitive accounts of creation stress the essential relationships of God and human persons, of human persons and others, and of human persons to the rest of the created world. The plan of creation implies interdependence as well as the need for each species to reproduce and multiply. Just as it was not good "for the man to be alone" (Gen 2:18), so, too, it is not possible for people to develop their full human and spiritual potential in isolation one from the other. If life is to be experienced in its plenitude, if human persons are to become what

God has intended, this will be accomplished through relationships. By God's plan, we are dependent upon him and mutually interdependent on one other for our fulfillment.

In this context sin can be understood as a willful refusal on the part of persons to acknowledge and respect these divinely ordained relationships, especially the bond that exists between God and his human creatures. Sin has a specific relevance inasmuch as it represents the interruption in the order to these relationships. Sin has immediate, widespread, and calamitous consequences, and these are depicted in the Genesis accounts. Sin creates a context in which more alienation and disintegration is inevitable. It distances one from God, distorts the understanding of the essential dependence of creature upon Creator, and disrupts the relationships that exist among people. It is seen on all significant levels of human life: the religious, social, intrapersonal, and even the cosmic. From this perspective one can understand why exaggerations, frustrations, and failures are so often found in sexual relationships.

For Christians, the ministry of Jesus Christ is understood as one of reconciliation, of repairing the ways in which sin has fractured the important relationships noted above which are constitutive of human fulfillment. By his human relationships, Jesus modeled the power of understanding, forgiveness, and love to heal and to make whole. All of this was accomplished by the plan of his Father, which the author of the fourth Gospel describes: "And the Word became flesh and came to dwell among us" (Jn 1:14). Jesus became man; through his human personality, he mediated the reconciling and health dimensions of his mission.

The Christian Church can draw understanding and inspiration for its mission not only from what Jesus taught, but also from how he related to a wide variety of persons. It is from a contemplative appreciation of how Jesus ministered to others that we grasp the mandate for mission that we now share. Much emphasis has been placed on interpretation of the message of Jesus; far less emphasis has been placed on an analysis of the ways in which he related to others. Theologians rarely become involved in reflection which attempts to understand the relationship of the sexuality of the person, Jesus, to the mission entrusted to him by the Father.

Neither the Scriptures nor the Western Christian tradition has acknowledged or emphasized the relationship between Jesus' sexuality and his relationships. Emphasis has traditionally been placed on reconciliation through the cross and resurrection, and the manifestation and extension of that reconciliation in the Church.

Some Views on Sexuality and Sexual Expression

Human sexuality is understood in various ways in our society and in our churches. It seems important to identify some of these divergent views since any of them might be significant in a pastoral relationship.

A pastoral-theological understanding which views human sexuality as the foundation of all relationships contrasts sharply with a definition of sexuality that is focused on genital involvement. The former can sometimes lead people to underestimate the societal and procreational aspects of human sexuality just as the latter view can suggest that persons who are not sexually active are not sexual.

Implicitly, others might define sexuality in terms of the partner's gender leading to labeling as heterosexual, homosexual, or bisexual. Sympathetic to Cartesian dualism, some see sexual activity as proper to the body (matter), while sexual nonpractice as related to the soul (spirit). Subjected to this categorization, human sexuality is debased, viewed as something hostile to the human spirit.

In a report entitled, "A Study of Issues Concerning Homosexuality" (1986), presented by an advisory committee of the Lutheran Church in America, the issue of sexuality was summarized in this way:

> Sexuality derived from this primary relationship to God expressed in baptism cannot be defined solely in terms of sexual practice. Indeed, it is both offensive and limiting to do so. Sexuality from this perspective emphasizes the place of

passion, affection, emotion in our relationship with God and with others. Finally, it suggests that genital contact ought to be contained with the context of a covenant, a relationship that reflects the trust, fidelity, and commitment we experience in our relationship with God.

Sexuality from this theological perspective emphasizes quality of relationship, not kind or quantity of sexual action, not gender of partner. (p. 36)

Sexuality and the Churches: Some Issues for the Pastor

The social and religious backgrounds proper to the churches are very significant for pastoral care. Our respective traditions account for many of the attitudes, convictions, judgments, and feelings found among pastors and their parishioners. These traditions are an essential element in many of the problems and challenges the churches face in the area of human sexuality. It is therefore important to assess the impact of our past on the way we think about sexuality, and how that thinking affects our ministries.

For many of us who grew up in social and religious traditions dominated by an understanding of sexuality defined in terms of prohibitions concerning sexual practice, our attitudes have been shaped significantly by these earlier learnings. We have come to judge ourselves and others in terms of these assimilated norms. Some of our fears and prejudices related to sexuality have their origin in these reinforced early learnings. We came to believe that the moral life is more concerned with what people do than with who they are. In terms of sexuality, most of us were taught what we could and could not do. We received little understanding for what it means that God created us as sexual beings so that we could be in relationship with him and with others. We were little helped to integrate a broader appreciation of human sexuality into our moral understanding.

We need to integrate a significant relationship dimension into our understanding of sexuality. This task will not be easy since it will require a rethinking of the procreational and behavioral emphasis many of us grew up with. The need to place our sexual ethic in a context of relationships will tend to give a more positive quality to moral norms and change the manner in which we understand and explain to others the place of sexuality in human life.

Another issue is that the strict sexual ethic common to many traditions leads to strong and often negative personal judgments. Our churches have approved sexual behavior only when it is properly marital, when it occurs between husband and wife, and have consistently condemned those sexual behaviors that are non-marital and extramarital. The catechetical literature, preaching, and penitential practices in the respective churches have communicated forcefully these strict requirements.

One result is that those who do not conform to these requirements are likely to be judged as personally bad. Only those who accept and live by the accepted sexual norms are considered good. This has led many to repress aspects of their sexuality. Others have assumed heavy burdens of guilt and self-depreciation due to their failure to comply with the sexual ethic. Some have chosen to live a double life: they maintain a public appearance of propriety while privately deviating from the expected standards. Others have decided that the strict ethic cannot command their respect and have consequently abandoned any religiously based moral norms.

In an attempt to respond to this situation, many churches counsel their members to hate the sin but love the sinner. This is a laudable attempt to distinguish behavior from a valued person, but it is not likely to succeed. One difficulty is theological: sin is not purely behavioral but is the response of the whole person. The Scriptures remind us that sin proceeds from the heart of a person (Mk 7:20–23). From this perspective hatred for the sin implies a judgment on the sinner. Another difficulty is practical. Many people know that they are classified as "sinners" and feel deeply the negative impact of this label. What comes across to them is not the love that is professed, but the condemnation and rejection that is implied. This is frequently the experience of homosexual persons.

Another stress that faces the churches results from the conflict between developments in the wider society and private practice. Victorian and Edwardian societies had to accommodate changes in social mores. The American society of the 1960s and 1970s experienced a sexual revolution. These periods of social adjustment are not always easy, nor are they without excessive reaction as people search for reasonable compromise.

A relational understanding of sexuality, personalistic currents in theology, the tensions imposed by judgment, and the impact of changing social mores have all challenged the traditional genital understanding of human sexuality. Even though these challenges seem to be moving in healthy and constructive directions, the churches have not been too willing to consider new interpretations or to seek new formulations of their teachings on sexuality.

Sexuality has a larger place in the moral life than the microscopic place which a restrictive emphasis on action dictates. A strongly held code morality unquestionably has a legitimate place in an ethical discussion of sexuality, but not the primary and exclusive role which some social and religious traditions have accorded them. For the most part, the major religious traditions hold firm to an act-centered morality and continue to frame moral injunctions in predominantly negative terms, with all the judgmental effects this approach often entails.

Society, the Churches, and the Issues of Homosexuality

One example, among others, pertains to society and the churches' attitudes toward homosexuality. Not only is there social and religious opposition to homosexual actions, but there is intolerance for homosexual persons. Contemporary American society has begun slowly to address the roots of its intolerance for homosexual persons. Some of this was catalyzed by the social phenomenon called "the gay movement," the history of which is symbolically related to the Stonewall riot of 1969. Police in New York City raided a gay bar in Greenwich Village. This was not an uncommon occurrence. Alleged police brutality and selective arrests were routine. Stonewall was a turning point in the resistance of homosexual persons. The patrons fought back, and their response marshaled the response of homosexual persons across America to stand up for their dignity and rights.

While society struggles to integrate homosexual persons into the mainstream of its life, guaranteeing them their rights and dignity, the churches have been less successful in signaling acceptance. Let's look at some examples, cited in *Good-Bye, I Love You* (1986) by Carol Lynn Pearson. The book is the story of a homosexual man, his wife and four children, and their struggles with their divided loves, the Mormon Church, and AIDS.

Carol Lynn, acknowledging her husband's homosexuality, considered how they might work out their problems within the Mormon community in which they lived in Utah. The following provides some insight into her perception of the dilemma.

> *No one would counsel me to endure, I knew that. If we did not pull off the miracle [help her husband change his sexual orientation], I would surely be encouraged to leave Gerald. And yet I would be judged. To many, a divorced woman, for whatever reason, is a failure. Why had I married such a man in the first place, people would wonder. Why hadn't I been able to snap him out of it? . . .*
>
> *Our community viewed homosexuality as evil and disgusting. I couldn't bear to have people talking about Gerald as if he were a monster. In all the praying I had done, I had felt strongly that Gerald was as much loved of God as I was. I did not feel that the answer was to banish him or to separate him from his children.*
>
> *If the worst happened and we ended our marriage, could we somehow still maintain a relationship? That would be hard to do here. Crushing judgments and shame would take their toll. When a young man in a nearby town was discovered to be a homosexual, his mother had taken it upon herself to call BYU [Brigham Young University] and have him expelled from school. She then called his place of employment and told them he was gay and should be fired. She called every subsequent place he worked and gave the same information. She told him, "I want you to repent, and I know the only way you'll repent is to be reduced to the gutter. That's what I pray for."*

*Another Mormon mother, discovering that her teenage
son had had homosexual encounters, did not speak to him
for three months or set a place for him at table. She was
arranging to place him in a foster home. (pp. 115–116)*

When Carol Lynn and Gerald moved from Utah to California, they became part of the Mormon community in Walnut
Creek. Gerald resisted becoming involved in the life of the
church. He explained his reluctance to have his oldest child
baptized:

*"I don't want to turn our children over to an organiza-
tion that will teach them to hate their father," he said.*

*"Gerald," I responded quickly, "you know that there is
no person or organization anywhere on this earth that could
teach your children to hate you. You know they love and
adore you, and they always will."*

"But the Church will tell them that I am evil."

*"Look, Gerald," I said. "I understand your feelings to-
ward the Church, but without it you wouldn't have developed into the person you are, or have the spiritual interests
you do. I think the Church has done a lot for you."*

*There were tears in Gerald's eyes when he answered me.
"That's the trouble, Blossom [an endearing name Gerald
called his wife]. I love the Church. And the Church detests
me. That's why it hurts so much." (pp. 120–121)*

Homophobia and Pastoral Approaches

The brief excerpts from *Good-Bye, I Love You* highlight the
feelings of alienation from the Church that some gay and lesbian
persons feel. In times of great need, they feel abandoned. To a
significant extent they may have internalized the churches' act-
centered moral teachings concerning sexuality and sexual practice, and judged themselves as unworthy of membership. It is
true that some gay men and lesbian woman leave communities
of faith because they perceive or experience the Church as
unwelcoming or rejecting.

Apart from the principles of ethics which norm its life,
some Christian communities may also be homophobic. Homo-

phobia is a term that describes generically the range of hostile reactions people may have to lesbians and gay men. The roots of homophobia are many. Social psychologists and others have attempted to understand the variables that influence a person's negative attitudes and prejudices toward lesbians and gays.

Many phobias have their origins in irrational fears. Some people fear heights, others are afraid to be with others in crowded places. Some fear spiders, elevators, or suspension bridges. The majority of other healthy persons do not perceive a serious threat when exposed to these objects or experiences. However, others became physically and emotionally paralyzed when confronted with the same objects or experiences.

Homophobia is more than hostile or negative reactions grounded in irrational fears. It also includes prejudices. Prejudice, as the Latin noun *praejudicium* denotes, means a preconceived opinion or feeling, positive or negative, formed before a person has knowledge, thought, or reason. Just as with phobic reactions, one can work to change the prejudice by helping to change how a person thinks about lesbians and gay men.

American society and many ecclesial communities have thought about homosexuality as depraved, pathological, immoral, dangerous to the social welfare, and evil. For a variety of social and religious reasons, homosexuality in our culture has been defined negatively. It is not our intention either to defend or challenge the validity of this definition or these judgments. It is sufficient to note that a large consensus of the American people, exposed to these judgments and affected by them, fear homosexuality and themselves express negative opinions and feelings about lesbian and gay persons. Because the AIDS pandemic is linked to sexual transmission—largely, though not exclusively, through male homosexual acts—a new wave of fears and prejudices toward gays has been engaged.

Behavioral scientists are captivated by the phenomenon that, given comparable social and religious exposure, some heterosexual people are fearful, negative, hostile, and aggressive toward homosexual persons, while others are positively accepting, tolerant, and responsive. We also know that people can express similar attitudes—positive or negative—for entirely different reasons. For example, in a religious congregation, a minister is judged favorably by a large number of the members. When polled about their favorable judgments, the congregation will be divided on the variables that contribute to their assessment of the minister. Some may like his physical appearance, others the manner and tone of his preaching, still others his personal approach to individuals. While sharing a consensus in their favorable judgment, they are divided on what informs their opinion.

It is important that pastors who intend to work with persons with AIDS—numbers of whom come from social groups that do not enjoy popular acceptance or support—reassess their own fears and prejudices. To do so, let us look at some relevant issues.

Homophobia and Personal Experience

The issues of human sexuality pose several challenges to effective pastoral care. It is problematic when we attempt to provide pastoral care to persons with AIDS, a large percentage of whom have acquired the life-threatening virus through sexual transmission. Furthermore, of that population, a significant number of persons with AIDS come from a group whose sexual orientation, lifestyle, and behaviors elicit unfavorable and hostile social responses, vocal disapproval, and condemnation from many religious traditions. Consciously or unconsciously, pastors' attitudes may reflect the prevailing social and religious negativism. It is incumbent upon ministers who desire to be helpful to these populations of persons, who may be the objects of social and religious discrimination, to consider their own attitudes toward sexuality, and to entertain changes in those attitudes as they deem appropriate.

While pursuing graduate theological education, I was enrolled in a course on the Church and Pastoral Care. A number of experiential learning opportunities were provided in this course. I attended three weekend retreats whose purpose was to confront the participants' phobias and prejudices to three distinct groups: chemically dependent persons, persons of color, and gays.

I recall my reluctance and apprehension as the weekend dealing with homosexuality approached. One of my classmates called and informed me that he was withdrawing from participation in the experience. The conference was arranged in a church-affiliated retreat center. All participants roomed with a person from the target population. On different weekends I shared a room with a heroin addict, a black man, and a gay man.

In the group process, we were initially asked to share our beliefs and feelings about homosexuality and homosexual persons. Many of the theological students and ministers who participated acknowledged that they had little prior experience with homosexual people. The fact that the participants elected to engage in such an experience made the group somewhat atypical inasmuch as everyone was open to changing attitudes.

Working intensively with a diverse population of gay persons, the negative stereotypes and feelings we may have had toward lesbians and gay men were subjected to new sources of information and experience. We came to understand that security in our own gender identity and comfort with our own sexual orientation allowed us to be open to other people with differing experiences of their sexuality. Many of us who participated in these weekend experiences identified within ourselves fears and prejudices of which we were unaware. For me, and I suspect for many others of my fellow learners, these brief but intensive encounters have changed my attitudes and have shaped important aspects of my ministry.

Raoul, twenty-nine years old, was raised in an affluent, staunchly Roman Catholic, Puerto Rican family. Raoul attended a private Jesuit secondary school, and continued his collegiate and professional education in law at Harvard. He remained in the northeast after he graduated from law school, and became an assistant district attorney.

In November 1986, Raoul was diagnosed with AIDS. He talks about his conversation with a Jesuit priest whom he went to see.

> *When I was in high school, I was fond of a scholastic (a Jesuit preparing for ordination) who taught me math at Colegio San Ignacio in Rio Piedras. During the intervening years, we exchanged greetings at Christmas, although I haven't seen him in a dozen years.*

My diagnosis with AIDS has frightened me. For the first time in my life, I am thinking about death. I have felt so confused and alone. As I was thinking about my situation, Father Aguero's name came to mind. I picked up the telephone, called his residence in New York, and arranged to fly down to visit him.

It was a pleasant reunion after so many years. Father Aguero was still involved in teaching math in a school in Manhattan. He retained the enthusiasm and dedication that I had experienced when he taught me in Puerto Rico. We chatted about family and friends back home, and did a lot of reminiscing. Then I told him the real reason for my visit.

He seemed paralyzed by the revelation that I was gay and that I had AIDS. His whole approach to me changed when I brought up these topics for discussion. He was anxious, clearly not knowing how to respond to me. The more I spoke about my promiscuous lifestyle, my fears for the future, and my sense of estrangement from the Catholic Church, the less able was Fr. Aguero to reply.

Many times he said, "Raoul, I don't know why you are telling me these things; I can't help you." He appealed to the fact that he was not experienced in these things, that he was a math teacher. I went to Fr. Aguero because he was a friend and a priest, not because he was a math teacher! He tried to reassure me, but it was not consoling. His body told me the whole story. When I mentioned the word AIDS he reactively pushed his chair back. From that moment, we lost eye contact with each other. Fr. Aguero kept looking toward the darkened window, peering into the vacant night.

It occurred to me that I had made a mistake seeking to consult with Fr. Aguero. He is clearly not comfortable with gay men, and is fearful of persons with AIDS. Leaving him that evening, he assured me of his prayers. As I returned on the plane to Boston, I felt an even greater distance from the Church of my youth. Even my old friend Fr. Aguero could not bridge that chasm. . . .

In his monograph entitled *AIDS: The Spiritual Dilemma* (1987), John Fortunato describes his experience:

The Church has not done well in helping us gay and lesbian people on our spiritual journeys. In its terror of sexuality, it has been singularly put off by those whose sexuality, by ontological chance, is remarkable in its different-ness. Gay people draw the Church's attention to a piece of itself it frequently wishes would go away. Yet, I am convinced that Christianity (which is not the same thing as the Church) can help us. I am forced by study and experience to conclude that the spirituality that Jesus embodied and taught—as well as we can know these things through those frustrating, convoluted, muddy media called Holy Scripture and Tradition—speaks to our situation powerfully.

We who are marginalized by society so often feel like "strangers in a strange land," treated hostilely, as we are, by people who are terrified of what we represent to them. And I am persuaded that Jesus, who knew from personal experience exactly how we feel, points us toward spiritual roots where we can find the kind of grounding we need in order to make our lives—in all their joys and sorrows—meaningful. And, of course, this experience of being alienated is not known uniquely by gay people (pp. 8–9).

Fortunato's characterization of the alienation and disaffection that many gay persons experience within the institutional Church is helpful. While acknowledging that Fortunato's thesis may be overgeneralized, it nonetheless challenges pastors to reevaluate how their attitudes and behaviors may be contributing to these reactions.

Symbols are an important part of the way in which we understand ourselves. They support our perceptions and our identities. For example, because we think of ourselves as intellectually curious, we might be more inclined to attend a concert of contemporary music than someone who does not apply the same label in his or her self-assessment.

For the same reasons, those of us who have been raised in religious traditions which endorse restrictiveness in their attitudes toward human sexuality and express condemnation of homosexuality might be more inclined to express unfavorable attitudes ourselves. This may be intensified for those of us who are ordained representatives of those traditions. Our roles and functions may predispose us to maintain closed and rejecting attitudes toward lesbian and gay people.

In the course of any attempts to alter personal attitudes, one needs to become better informed. Reading and discussion in the areas of human sexuality and homosexuality are constructive. Appropriate reading in the expanding biological and psychological literature on these topics is a non-threatening and beneficial response to the need to know. There are many continuing education courses in human sexuality offered in major universities. Professionals and clergy frequently are participants in these experiences, and they bring a valued perspective to the discussions.

Religious ideologies can color the ways in which a person views his or her professional responsibilities. For example, persons who wear the uniform of a branch of the armed services of the United States may believe that they are obligated to defend affirmatively a particular foreign policy decision of the government. This belief may be rooted in their judgment that the symbol of the military uniform they wear requires conformity in thinking and behavior. This example is not meant to indict either the thinking or the behavior among those who guard and defend the national interests of the people of the United States, but simply to suggest that the symbol of a military uniform can influence the attitudes and behavior of the person who wears it.

There have been many priests who acknowledge that certain of their behaviors are modified when they are dressed in clerical garb. In these instances, their symbolic identification with ecclesial communities and religious traditions color their verbal behaviors and actions.

For attitudes to change, people need to enlarge their understandings of the symbol. If the symbolic meaning is very restricted, it might need to be broadened. Clergy can benefit from the example of others who broaden the symbol. For example, a Catholic bishop who sets aside a certain amount of time on a regular basis to provide basic physical care for hospitalized persons with AIDS may be an important symbol to other priests in his diocese. It may communicate that it is desirable that the Church become identified more visibly with persons with AIDS, apart from doctrinal, moral, or ideological positions on sexuality and practice.

Becoming involved in the care for persons with AIDS, especially gay men, helps enormously to change the attitudes and stereotypes that one may have concerning sexuality in general, and homosexuality in particular. Ministerial formation programs in the area of clinical pastoral education provide many opportunities for experiential encounters that precipitate confrontations with one's attitudes. When appropriate changes take place, there is a concomitant reduction in anxiety in contacts that involve issues of sexuality, and a relaxation in the defensive postures that often detract from effective pastoral care.

DEATH

Death and Society

For many people, AIDS means death. The primary meaning of Acquired Immunodeficiency Syndrome is that the body's defenses are so weakened that one's very life is threatened. The popular understanding of AIDS is that it is a terminal disease, for which, at present, there is no cure. AIDS bears the stigma of death.

Concerns with mortality have captivated the fantasies and fears of many people throughout human history. Some have characterized modern medicine not so much in terms of its health maintenance functions as in terms of its efforts to control death. A basic fact of human life is that it is finite. Consciousness of mortality gives greater definition, meaning, and purpose to the time available for living. For some religious traditions, the fact of death symbolizes the transition to a fuller experience of life. The awareness of death, therefore, can have beneficial influences on human development and response.

Persons with terminal diagnoses often report that they begin to see their remaining life with a different meaning and purpose. They often assign different values and priorities to aspects of their life, and make important choices and decisions.

They admit some people to greater intimacy, and exclude others. The approach of death catalyzes the process of integration of values and experiences. However, the fact that human finitude and physical death have developmental significance does not mitigate the anxieties that some people experience when confronted with the prospect of death.

If death were a logical and predictable event in human life, some might find it more easy to prepare for it, and to accept its inevitable timetable. As we know, death is not subject to these restraints of logic and temporal schedule. Nonetheless, many of us live with the reasonable anticipation of a long life. When death occurs earlier in the life course, this can be disturbing to survivors who are reminded of our inability to control certain dimensions of our own mortality.

AIDS has reinforced the destabilizing realization that human life is vulnerable and survival is compromised. A fragile virus which imperceptibly enters the human body can threaten the very immune system functions whose purposes are to defend the body's life. Although the virus has no regard for sex, age, or race, it has infected significant numbers of otherwise healthy and vital young men and women, a large percentage of whom have died or are dying.

Our society has provided compelling evidence of its discomfort with death. Some social scientists have labeled us a death-denying and death-defying people. We protect ourselves from conscious acknowledgement of our mortality. Our behavior on the nation's highways which places our lives and those of others in jeopardy, our habits of overeating, and our abusive involvement with alcohol and other drugs support the thesis that Americans act as if they were immortal. We bolster these beliefs by thinking that the cars we drive are safe and that we can medically or surgically correct any damage caused by obesity or substance abuse.

American society does everything it can to shelter and protect individuals from the signs, symbols, and experiences of death. While emphasizing the culture of youthfulness, we deny the realities of aging and mortality. Our society is content when the elderly segregate in communities apart from the others. There is a comfort when older people accept to live out their final days in nursing homes. There is relief when a loved one acquiesces to die in a hospital or a residential hospice. The funeral industry supports our denial of death by striving to achieve cosmetic illusions of vitality with the cadavers they display. Death is disguised and mourning rituals are devalued and trivialized. Many find it difficult to talk with comfort to bereaved individuals. It is much easier to avoid the subject, to treat death as if it didn't happen.

Medical and nursing practice reinforce these cultural attitudes and biases toward death. Our technological advances, particularly in medical diagnosis and treatment, have been able to isolate and treat so many life-threatening conditions that many of us are conditioned to believe that we can, in fact, conquer most of the enemies that challenge human life and survival. We feel we are in control of our lives.

The pandemic of AIDS is unsettling on the social level because it blatantly confronts the postures of defiance and denial vis-à-vis death. By its very definition, AIDS is described as disabling the body's natural defenses. Because AIDS is a serious international health threat, the World Health Organization in 1987 committed itself to global prevention and control. Efforts like this bring the threat to survival to the level of consciousness. Society is forced to face the dangers, while at the same time acknowledging its limitations in treating infected persons, and its present inability to cure the disease. Society is confronted with the realization that AIDS kills. The number of persons with AIDS continues to increase and the statistics of those who die as a result of AIDS-related illnesses steadily mount.

The Humanization of Death

American society may be characterized as death-denying and death defying, but this does not imply that our culture is insensitive and unresponsive to dying persons. Over the course of the last twenty years, there has been movement and change in our corporate attitudes toward death and dying. Through reading, academic courses, and discussions, Americans have attempted to explore their own feelings and fears about death.

Health care professionals recognize the importance and benefits of acquiring the understanding and skills necessary to work effectively with the dying. Medicine and nursing, often seen as symbolic frontline troops in the war against disease and death, acknowledge that while they are better able to sustain life, they are unable to defeat death. Helping a person to die is as much a part of the practice of medicine and nursing as helping a person to live.

Effective human care of the dying is contingent upon the integration of personal mortality into one's personality and outlook. Those who work with dying persons and their families must make peace with the finitude of human life. When individuals do not come to terms with this basic fact of life, not only on an intellectual level, but on the level of feelings as well, then they are in danger of doing harm to dying persons in their care. When a personal confrontation with death is not accepted or dealt with effectively by health care professionals, they become especially vulnerable to feelings of inadequacy, anger, guilt, helplessness, or frustrations as they attempt to care for a terminally ill person.

The humanization of death means allowing the defenses to relax sufficiently so that the fact of death can take its place in the comprehensive understanding of human life. Death requires its legitimate place in human development. Not to attempt to locate its meaning is to subject oneself to needless anxieties and debilitating fears.

Death and Pastoral Care

When we think about religious professionals and death, we may assume falsely that all clergy are comfortable with the realities of death. Since many traditions hold firm to a faith in an afterlife, death is interpreted as a transition point to a fuller life. The Roman Catholic ritual asserts that "life is not ended, merely changed." Many religious traditions speak affirmatively about death as the fulfillment of human life. Theologies support an understanding of the immortality of the human soul, the eternal survival of the spirit.

Despite scriptural, doctrinal, and traditional evidence that undergirds positive and comforting approaches to death in many religious sects, this does not mean that all persons adhering to a particular religious faith are comfortable with death. This is certainly not true of all clergy who are leaders within these various denominations.

Like health care professionals, clergy have their own anxieties and fears associated with death and dying persons. They are the products of the social environments in which they have lived and in which they were educated. Seminaries charged by the various religious groups to provide theological education for clergy, like medical and nursing programs, recognize the importance of death education, but rarely is this an integral part of their requirements. Clinical pastoral programs provide seminarians and ordained clergy with greater opportunities for acquiring experiential learning in the care of dying persons, but a large percentage of clergy have not profited from such experiences. Many men and women are ordained for ministerial service with no direct experiences or acquired skills in interacting with dying persons. Yet, their ministry requires that they be present and assist the dying and their families.

One of the more problematic issues of clergy who have not come to terms with personal mortality is their avoidance of or emotional distancing from persons who are terminally ill. It is understandable that people instinctively defend themselves from those things they perceive as threatening. Just as society can avoid involvements with older, handicapped, drug-dependent, and terminally ill persons, clergy can similarly disengage. It is not ethical for physicians to deny care to any person in need. It is similarly unethical for clergy to deny pastoral assistance to any person desirous of support. However, the quality of care may be compromised in both instances by the conscious or unconscious attitudes of the care providers.

Many clergy vigorously deny that they have any fears about death. They marshal all the tenets of their religious traditions to support their beliefs about death and life. They cite all their experiences in presiding at funerals of parishioners and their many pastoral visitations to hospitals and nursing homes. And yet, for some of these widely experienced clergy, there is apparent discomfort with dying persons.

Discomfort may be intensified for clergy when the dying person belongs to certain age or disease groups. For example, many health care professionals acknowledge difficulties in assisting terminally ill children and their families. Others comment on difficulties in caring for individuals who have been disfigured as a result of disease or accident. Finally, there may be problems for some in attending individuals who have been directly responsible for their life-threatening condition, for example, a person who is critically ill as a result of a drug overdose. Clergy may experience comparable problems when they interact with similar populations of terminally ill persons. Persons with AIDS are a new population that is added to the roster of difficult cases.

The majority of people dying with AIDS tend to be drawn from cohorts of younger persons. Secondly, they tend to develop multiple infections over the course of an extended period of time, which require repeated hospitalizations and aggressive drug treatments. The disease and its treatments can severely alter body structure, including weight and hair loss, discoloration, and disfiguring lesions. Finally, in many cases, lifestyle choices may have directly or indirectly contributed to a person's exposure to the AIDS virus. In this sense, blame for the disease may be implied. It is not uncommon to hear personnel in hospitals which care for persons with AIDS comment, "It's tragic, but they brought it on themselves."

Kevin McNulty had grown up in a neighborhood which was predominantly middle-class Irish American and Roman Catholic. Much of the community's life was centered around the parish church. All of the youth activities within the neighborhood were church-sponsored. Kevin belonged to many of these youth groups, and continued to assist as a young adult leader while he was in college. After graduation he accepted a job which required that he relocate to New York City.

Three years later, at age twenty-five, Kevin developed a serious case of Cytomegalovirus. The infection affected his eyesight. He also developed pneumonia. While being treated for CMV, Kevin's mouth became involved with yeast infections; white plaques began to proliferate in his mouth, spreading into his esophagus and lungs. Coupled with swollen lymph glands, it was uncomfortable for Kevin to swallow.

Kevin's parents insisted that he be transferred to a Boston hospital so that he would be close to family who could care for him. While hospitalized, he was visited by Fr. Hamilton, a priest with whom he formerly had worked in some of the parish youth programs. Kevin's parents had requested the visit, having confided to Fr. Hamilton that Kevin was gay and that he had AIDS. At the time of the visit, Kevin was seriously ill, but not in imminent danger of death.

Fr. Hamilton entered Kevin's room at Massachusetts General Hospital with some evident discomfort. He had never spoken to Kevin about his homosexuality, and did not know if he should raise this topic with Kevin. His discomfort was masked by his "business as usual" approach. Kevin's eyes began to tear as the priest entered his room. His parents who were also visiting left the room so that Kevin and Fr. Hamilton could visit alone.

Kevin was aware that his parents had spoken previously to Fr. Hamilton and that the priest had been briefed confidentially about Kevin's diagnosis and background. Kevin was actually relieved to know that his parents had provided these background data.

Fr. Hamilton began to speak about the youth group activities of the parish. He was animated as he described a number of recent events, commenting on the people with whom he works, some of whom Kevin knew. Kevin tried to remain engaged as the priest continued speaking. At a point, Kevin said, "Father, I'm afraid that I'm not going to make it. I think I'm going to die of this thing." Fr. Hamilton was surprised at the directness of Kevin's statement.

"Kevin, you are in very competent hands here at Massachusetts General. They're going to help you get well. Don't despair! Where's the 'dig-in determination' of the guy who used to play shortstop for Saint Aidan's baseball team?" As Kevin listened to the priest's attempts to encourage and reassure him, he felt very ambivalent. On the one hand, he felt comforted that his parish priest had come to visit and support him. On the other hand, he was frustrated that the priest seemed to be avoiding the real concerns Kevin had about dying. It seemed that the priest didn't want to deal with the fact that Kevin was gay (something Kevin knew the priest disapproved), and that he was gravely ill with AIDS. As a result, Kevin felt alone. He thought that Fr. Hamilton would be a person to whom he could open his heart. As the visit progressed, Kevin began to realize that Fr. Hamilton did not seem able to deal with his pressing concerns about death. The most Fr. Hamilton could say was "Kevin, you've got to fight, put some weight back on, and regain your will to go on living."

Kevin never lost the will to live. After a lingering illness, including two more hospitalizations, Kevin died in his parents' home, fifteen months after his initial diagnosis. Fr. Hamilton remained in contact during these months, but Kevin and he never found a comfortable common ground of sharing.

This case reveals the problems some clergy have in dealing with a young person with AIDS. The story was related by Kevin's mother who became her son's closest human support through the course of his final illness. It was Kevin who shared this experience with her. Mrs. McNulty was disappointed that a priest would be unable to accept the reality that a young man was dying of AIDS. She said, "We knew he understood how sick Kevin was, because he discussed it many times with us. But he was not able to connect with Kevin. In the end, Kevin didn't really want to see him, although Fr. Hamilton kept coming. Sometimes I had to make excuses to respect Kevin's wishes."

We do not know what Fr. Hamilton experienced since he was not interviewed. Many clergy involved in pastoral work with dying persons, including persons with AIDS, admit that they feel impotent in face of the overwhelming psychological and spiritual needs of the dying. Fr. Hamilton may have experienced some of these things in his attempts to minister to Kevin. He seemed emotionally unable to accept the reality of Kevin's life-threatening illness, and his progressive deterioration. His frequent comments about Kevin's emaciated appearance and lack of energy betrayed his discomfort with the signs of Kevin's waning hold on life. From the first communication by his parents about Kevin's homosexuality, Fr. Hamilton never raised the subject again. His silence may have signaled that he was not willing or able to respond to this issue. The McNultys overcame their fears and negative biases, and were wonderfully supportive of their son and brother during his difficult ordeal. Fr. Hamilton, on the contrary, always remained on the periphery, and never succeeded in providing the kind of companionship Kevin needed in his final journey.

5

Pastoral Care and the Psychosocial Needs of Persons with AIDS

Early in the Gospel of Mark (1:40–45), there is a narrative account of a meeting between Jesus and a man afflicted with leprosy. In the Jewish society of Jesus' day, leprosy was the ultimate form of uncleanness. Lepers were excluded from participation in the community. They were thought to be a source of defilement for others.

In the Marcan story, the leper approached Jesus and begged, "If you will, you can make me clean." The evangelist focuses on the reaction of Jesus. Many texts translate Jesus' emotional response as "moved with pity." However, many commentators note that the more accurate rendition of Jesus' reaction is, "moved with anger." This latter translation is perhaps more authentic. When Jesus was confronted with a person whose illness had excommunicated him from others, he felt anger and indignation. The leper brought Jesus face to face with the powers of evil.

The emotional response of Jesus, the sense of injustice he felt at the leper's social isolation, interpret his subsequent actions. The Gospel writer tells us that Jesus touched him, a most unlikely thing since it meant Jesus himself was defiled by that physical contact. It is a gesture of acceptance, of support, of solidarity with the afflicted. By that gesture, the text observes that the leprosy "left" him, as if the power of evil departed from him. Jesus' physical gesture of touch and his words helped restore the man to a rightful place in the community. Emphasis is not placed on the healing act itself, but on the understanding, compassion, indignation, and reconciliation of Jesus.

Providing pastoral care for a person with AIDS is a parallel situation to the scenario in Mark's Gospel. Some have referred to AIDS as the modern leprosy. To be effective in the ministry to persons with AIDS requires that, like Jesus, we feel "moved with anger." We need to feel the social and psychological isolation of persons with AIDS, the ways in which they are separated from community supports. In AIDS, we come face to face with evil.

To be able to minister effectively to this new group of contemporary lepers requires a variety of helping skills. One of these skills involves making a competent assessment of the psychosocial strengths and weaknesses of the person being helped. While this is an integral part of medical and nursing education, it has not always been a component of pastoral education. In this chapter we shall consider some of the psychosocial issues to which pastors should be sensitive when offering their assistance to persons with AIDS. While it is clear that persons with AIDS or ARC have physical stresses related to weakened body immunity, one should not assume that there is a parallel weakness in psychological functioning.

Primary Contact

The initial contact with a person with AIDS is important, both for the individual and for the pastor. For the person with AIDS, it represents either the establishment, reconnection, or continuation of relationship with a community of faith. For the pastor, it provides an occasion in which to reach out, to "touch" a person. This means to establish rapport, trust, and confidence, as well as to begin to assess what will be required in pastoral care.

As in any effort to help another person—whether it is in counseling, psychotherapy, or pastoral care—a common goal is to assist an individual to make maximum use of the resources at his or her disposal. The Church has a repertory of resources that may assist an individual in need. It is important that the proper resources be selected and utilized. Some pastors prematurely select resources they judge to be helpful, only to discover that the individual is indifferent, non-responsive, or rejecting of such ministries. In some cases, the resources the pastor selects are disturbing, counterproductive, or damaging to the person in need.

For priests and other ministers whose religious tradition depends heavily upon the administration of sacraments as the foundation of pastoral care, this is particularly important. Within this context, a pastor may be inclined to begin a relationship by "doing" something, rather than taking the essential time to establish a relationship, make a competent assessment of the person's needs, and then begin to help the individual choose the appropriate resources in order to respond to these needs. The following case, which we shall analyze in some depth, exemplifies the "doing" strategy of pastoral care.

David, thirty-seven years old, had been living alone in San Francisco when he was diagnosed with Pneumocystis carinii pneumonia. He was treated at San Francisco General Hospital, and returned to work as a corporate attorney. Shortly after his return to his law practice, his health began to deteriorate to such a degree that he required home-care assistance. His brother and sister-in-law from Connecticut offered to take care of him in their home. After consideration of many issues, including opportunities for medical care, separation from friends, and distance from his law practice, David elected to accept his family's invitation.

During a subsequent hospitalization in Connecticut for a recurrent PCP infection, David was visited by a Catholic priest. Baptized and raised in the Roman Catholic faith, David had been a non-practicing, nominal Catholic since he entered college. Because David had noted on his admission record his religious affiliation as "Catholic" and since his medical condition was grave, he was automatically visited by the Catholic chaplain.

Upon entering his room, the chaplain was attired in his habit and wore a purple stole around his neck. He was friendly and jovial. After a few opening remarks, he announced: "Well, David, let's get a few things straight with the Lord. I'll hear your confession and then give you the sacrament of the sick. Now how long has it been since your last confession, son?"

David was clearly stunned and agitated by the priest's approach to him, but he was not strong enough physically to confront him. He simply said, "Father, could we do this some other time?" The priest said: "No bother, son. Just make a good act of contrition and I'll give you absolution." With that he raced through some scarcely audible prayers while anointing David's forehead and hands. David lay motionless in the bed. As he concluded, the priest smiled and made some light comment and departed waving a farewell blessing.

The initial contact in many cases colors the subsequent relationship and the potential effectiveness of the one offering care. Although the chaplain who attempted to minister to David was a caring individual, he was negligent and inattentive to the essential elements of a helping relationship. He took no time to assess David's needs, elicit his desires, and respect his requests. Even when David was able to suggest that he needed more time to sort out whether and how he might desire to be reconciled with the Catholic Church, the priest proceeded to accomplish his own agenda, namely to administer the sacraments.

Because the priest's philosophical and theological education stressed the essential and inherent value of this form of ministry to persons in need, the chaplain left David's room with a certain sense of accomplishment. When one applies a different set of criteria to pastoral ministry, it is easy to see how one could judge the intervention to be not only ineffective, but potentially further alienating to the sick person.

What is suggested here is that taking the time to attend to the establishment of a relationship with the person with AIDS is an indispensable prerequisite to any effective pastoral care ministry. The "Who are you?" and "What do you need?" questions are indispensable. The formation of an accepting and understanding relationship makes it possible for the pastor to begin assessing the person's psychosocial resources. Let's turn our attention to some specific areas a pastor may wish to explore.

The Individual's Perception of His/Her Illness

A person with AIDS may have experience with the disease antedating his or her diagnosis. Because AIDS has been prevalent in certain populations identified early as high-risk groups (for example, among gay men and IV drug users), many people have first-hand knowledge and experience about the syndrome. Knowledge, however, is variable, and a person's perceptions of the disease vary.

When David was first diagnosed in 1985, he responded quickly to intravenous Trimethoprim treatment. His hospitalization was brief, and he was able to resume work quickly, while returning to the hospital to complete his program. Although he understood he had AIDS, he interpreted his quick response to treatment to mean that he was more healthy than other persons with AIDS. In fact, his general health and lifestyle were better than many other PCP patients.

He was not prepared for the subsequent deterioration of his health and his inability to work and care for himself. Certainly he did not anticipate that he would require the assistance of his brother and family in Connecticut. When hospitalized for recurrent PCP infection, David was unwilling to acknowledge how life-threatening was his relapse.

It is essential to know how David understands his condition and how much he is able or willing to do. A pastor requires a basic knowledge of the person's perception of his or her illness.

General Psychological Functioning

When the priest first entered David's room, he was lying in his bed, staring at the ceiling. He appeared motionless and weak. His mood was depressed. Although his family has been supportive and visited every day, he felt alone. All of his significant friends were in San Francisco. He received notes, cards, and some telephone calls from several of them. Two of the attorneys in his firm visited him in the hospital while they were on business trips to New York.

David's depression is related to his perceived isolation and his deteriorating physical health. He lacks a relationship with someone with whom he can begin to verbalize the feelings he is processing within. Although the doctors caring for him in the Connecticut hospital are empathic, he has not been able to open up to any of them on a significant level. This is not an uncommon situation with persons with AIDS. Concerned about providing complex medical services, the psychosocial needs of a patient may be neglected by some health care providers. A skilled pastor can respond to this deficit in care.

Fortunately, neither the disease nor the drug treatments have impaired seriously David's cognitive abilities. He thinks about himself and his future constantly, is preoccupied with many details, but has not been able to express many of these concerns. In practice, most persons with AIDS and ARC do adjust to their diagnoses and life-threatening diseases, and do not develop extraordinary psychosocial problems. It is the experience of many individuals who work with persons with AIDS to discover that these individuals are positively committed to living a quality life until they die. Persons with AIDS make decisions in light of this goal of living. However, they do need understanding and support to realize these objectives.

The priest's approach to David was abrupt and intrusive. He did not take sufficient time to get to know David and his psychological and spiritual status. The pastor did not correctly assess his affect and mood. As a result what he proposed to do was precipitous and unhelpful. David may have welcomed an opportunity "to confess," to open himself up to someone who could listen and respond, but he soon concluded that this priest would not be that person.

Stress

Coping with a life-threatening illness is inherently stressful. Stress is evident on the level of the disease and physical care. Stress is defined as a person's psychological and bodily responses to demands that either approach or exceed the limits of his or her coping abilities. Because of the nature of opportunistic infections and immunodeficiency, a person with AIDS lives with the ever-present possibility of a new threat or a new medical crisis, often occurring before the body has been able to recuperate or detoxify from earlier physical battles. This is a major source of stress for persons with ARC or AIDS.

Stress also is evident on many levels of psychological functioning. How a person perceives, interprets, and understands the environment in which he or she is situated determines to a great extent the degree of stress and anxiety he or she will experience. Life situations present a person with information and provide the necessary feedback for forming an understanding of the world. We rely heavily on these sources of data. Our behavioral responses are understood in relation to these situational conditions. Behavior does not exist in isolation from real life situations.

Some persons are more vulnerable than others to the physical and psychological stressors associated with a diagnosis of AIDS. Stress and anxiety are not synonymous. Anxiety always involves stress, but the reverse is not necessarily true. A diagnosis of AIDS, for example, may lead to stress, but not necessarily to anxiety. Which stressors lead to stress depends upon the person's assessment of them as threatening in some sense. Although many people like to separate the physical and psychological dimensions of stress, they are related. How a person selects, perceives, interprets, and uses information from a certain situation will influence how he or she reacts to it emotionally and physiologically.

Let's return to our case study to demonstrate how David is experiencing stress.

Until his first hospitalization, David had been a very healthy and athletic man. Although his professional work was demanding, David took appropriate time for leisure and recreation, and managed well his stresses. The diagnosis of Pneumocystis carinii pneumonia, while frightening, was manageable. As noted before, David was encouraged by his relatively quick recovery from his first infection.

When David had to decide whether to remain in San Francisco or accept his brother's invitation to be closer to family while accessible to competent medical care, the psychological stresses he experienced were significant.

He did not have a close relationship with his brother and sister-in-law. Although they were genuine, appropriate, and caring in their response to him, he knew that they were uncomfortable with the knowledge of his homosexuality and his AIDS diagnosis. Being in their large home was not comfortable, although he did have some measure of privacy. The transition, in this respect, was perceived as stressful.

When he was hospitalized again for a recurrent PCP infection, David continued to experience stress. Like many seriously ill individuals, David felt that he was losing control over his life. If there is anything that persons with AIDS resent strongly, it is being termed "victims." And yet, this is precisely what AIDS attempts to do. In his case, a thirty-seven year old bright, successful attorney who was in charge of his life now senses that it has been abruptly taken out of his control.

As David lies in his hospital bed in Connecticut, gazing at the ceiling, he is pondering these multiple experiences. He is processing his perceptions and interpretations. How he understands the total environment accounts for the psychological stress he is feeling. He is concerned whether his shortness of breath and low energy means that the Pneumocystis is unresponsive to treatment. He muses whether the corporation for which he works will decide to terminate him. He is concerned about the stresses and burdens he is placing on his brother and his family, the anxiety he senses in their home, and the stigma they may be experiencing by having a person with AIDS in their household. He already knows the disruption and inconvenience he has caused in their lives since he returned to Connecticut. While he is appreciative of their love and support, he also resents the way his brother patronizes him, making him feel less in charge of his own life. He has been unable to express much of this to his brother and sister-in-law.

The present and the uncertain future are not the only stressors that David feels. He is also stressed by his past memories. As he reviews his earlier life and searches his own behaviors looking for the ways in which he might have been infected by the virus, some of these memories are disquieting. He had never lived in a long-term relationship, but had a number of transient homosexual relationships. Although he had friends in the gay community in San Francisco, he did not participate actively. He had not talked openly about his homosexuality, and found now that he had much to process. All of this was experienced as stress.

Pastoral care is one vehicle for assisting David to manage some of these sources of stress. To do so, a pastor must have a clear understanding of what these issues are, and how much and how willing David is to explore these concerns. Pastors can do some practical things to help a person manage stress. Let me review some basic strategies which any pastor can utilize.

The first has to do with a simple recognition and acceptance that the person's situation is stressful. In David's case, it means accepting the fact that it is difficult for a successful person with a promising future to have contracted a life-threatening illness which has necessitated a return to his family's care. And the prospect is that things will continue to be stressful. A recognition and rehearsal of these "facts" helps a person to plan preparatory actions to deal with subsequent crises. There is a lot people can do to manage stress; it begins with an acceptance of vulnerability, and a commitment to plan for dealing with the sources of stress.

The second thing a pastor can do for a person like David is to begin to work with the feelings of helplessness, hopelessness, and demoralization by emphasizing the reassuring facts about personal and social coping resources. We talked about some of these issues in the earlier chapter on hope. A person can be assisted to feel reasonably confident that he or she has the resources to face the current situation and manage well. Persons with AIDS can manage to live in spite of the serious physical, psychological, and spiritual threats they may feel.

And, finally, a pastor can encourage a person like David to work out his own ways of reassuring himself and formulating his own plans for protecting himself from the stressors he is confronting. David was already showing signs of becoming passive and overly dependent upon his brother, other members of his family, and the physicians who were caring for him. He needs help to rebuild his cognitive defenses, to regain a sense of self-reliance. A pastor can help him to regain these sources of independence so that he does not rely exclusively on others to protect him from the suffering and losses associated with AIDS.

In doing these things, a pastor needs to strike a balance between the arousal of anticipatory grief and fear on the one hand, and realistic hope and genuine reassurance on the other. Some people can deal well with facing reality; others cannot. A pastor needs to be able to recognize the difference. In any case, it is important to assess the perceived areas of stress, and to make a determination of what might be appropriate to address and on what timetable.

Stigma

A person with AIDS is stigmatized. When we speak about stigma, we refer to the ways in which society deals with undesirable differentness. In classical Hellenic Greek, the word *stigma* meant an actual physical mark, cut or burned into a person's skin, designating the individual's particular defect. By this bodily sign, the rest of society could recognize the identity of the disgraced, infamous, or flawed person and avoid contact with such undesirable people.

In the Christian era, the term *stigma* acquired a level of religious meaning. Some of the saints had bodily eruptions which were interpreted as a divine sign of their special holiness. The *stigmata* or the lesions on the hands and feet of Francis of Assisi were interpreted as indications of God's favor. In other persons, physical abnormalities or diseases were interpreted as signs of God's disfavor. The favorable and unfavorable religious meanings attributed to these various signs demonstrate the cultural relativism accruing to stigmas.

In practice in America today, a person who is stigmatized is perceived as abnormal and deviant, and in some instances is dehumanized. The association of stigma with religious experience has been lost. A person who is stigmatized in our society is marginated, set apart from others. People treat the individual as dangerous, untrustworthy, objectionable. The person is not considered a fit member of society. And the impact of stigma extends beyond the people so marked. It affects the person's family, friends, and business associates, as well as those professionals who are involved with the stigmatized individual.

Many persons included in the high-risk groups for AIDS bear stigma labels apart from their infection with HIV. Terms such as junkies, druggies, whores, faggots and queers symbolize the stigmatization of each of these so-called socially deviant groups. Although AIDS is a syndrome of diseases, the acronym has become a new stigma label. Persons with AIDS are legitimately afraid that others will learn of their diagnosis, realizing that they will be stigmatized further if such knowledge is communicated.

For the pastor initiating ministry to a person with AIDS these issues have immediate relevance. A pastor will recognize the emotional effects of stigma. A person with AIDS often feels unclean, despicable, unworthy. Although AIDS is not easily transmitted, certainly not in ordinary non-sexual contact, some persons with AIDS feel that others think they are contagious, and thus to be avoided. A person with AIDS may be embarrassed to face the pastor, fearing that they will be judged as deserving of their fate. How many in our society, including religious leaders, have suggested that AIDS is God's vengeance on depraved persons? Stigmatization is emotionally scarring; it victimizes the person so branded.

It is very important that a pastor recognize, acknowledge, and respond to the personal apprehension, frustrations, and tensions associated with the stigma of an AIDS diagnosis. Pastoral care must encompass the family and friends whose lives are also affected by the stigma of AIDS. As health care workers have experienced stigma because of their work with persons with AIDS, so pastors must be prepared for the negative effect associated with our AIDS-related ministries.

Stigma can be reduced by education and modeling. As pastors we can do much to confront the attitudes, misinformation, and prejudices associated with this disease and the individuals who have become infected. The quality of our interpersonal relationships with persons with AIDS will help to neutralize the negative effects of the stigma associated with this disease. As trusted leaders within our local communities, pastors can do much to confront the injustices associated with the growing stigmatization of persons with AIDS and their families.

Communication

Whenever human beings interact, communication is operating on a variety of levels. The most obvious level is when plain, direct words are exchanged. Another level involves non-verbal language, particularly body posture, gestures, and facial movements. And, finally, there is symbolic, verbal language. The images we select, poetry we recall, and jokes we tell all carry important messages.

Too many of us limit what we receive in communication from another to the first level: plain language. Even then we may not listen effectively to that message. When the chaplain entered David's room and began his prologue to anointing, David said in a quiet whisper: "Father, could we do this some other time?" But there are many non-verbal cues that provide useful information about an individual's psychological and spiritual adjustment.

Non-verbalized feelings are defined as emotions or feelings which an individual may not be able to express in words, but which are being communicated nonetheless, even though the person may be unaware that they are being transmitted. Physical behaviors, facial expressions, gestures, and postures are all important sources of communication of feelings. How to interpret accurately the meaning of these non-verbal cues is an important but difficult task of the pastor in ministering to a person with AIDS.

What was David's behavior trying to communicate? Minimally, we would understand that he was unprepared for what the priest had proposed to do. His body resisted the approach. We could also infer from his direct words that he might be open to the priest's invitation at some later time, when David himself might be better in control of the situation. It is distressing that the chaplain did not grasp these most basic verbal and non-verbal cues in David's request. The chaplain assumed fatigue and reduced the requirements for reception of the sacraments. He proceeded to attend to his own agenda, namely, the administration of the sacraments. David, having been misunderstood and too weak to assert himself further, acquiesced to the priest's control.

If we can picture David lying in the bed, staring at the ceiling, we may be able to interpret this non-verbal communication. We may understand from this that he is preoccupied with a number of issues. We might also understand how the priest's sudden intrusion has startled him. Without taking the time to introduce himself by name, the priest made an abrupt transition to performing religious rituals. The priest failed to correctly interpret David's agitation. Although David's voice is weak, if we listened closely enough we could perceive the resistance and annoyance in his intonation, while he struggles to maintain proper respect for the good intentioned behavior of the priest.

Supportive pastoral care depends upon effective, mutual communication. The sensitive pastor must make an assessment of all the ways in which the person with AIDS is attempting to communicate. Non-verbalized feelings are an important component of human communication. They are the only reasonable alternative to spoken communication. Many people in life-threatening situations rely heavily on this latter form of communication. A comprehensive understanding of a person's needs and behavior is often contingent upon a correct assessment of the non-verbal cues and feelings. Correctly interpreting these various strata of communication will assist greatly in strategizing how best to respond to the messages being received.

Basic Psychological Needs:
Safety, Trust, Security

A life-threatening disease can be experienced by the ill individual as physically and emotionally destabilizing. The physical aspects of an illness and the program used to treat it can overtax a person's energy reserves. Serious illness is also an emotional strain. It is important to be able to assess how the experience of illness is affecting a person's basic functioning, particularly psychological activities.

At the bedrock of healthy psychological functioning are issues of safety, trust, and security. While these three basic needs are crucial for a child's psychological development, they continue to be important for adult functioning, particularly when a person is faced with the threat of serious illness. Illness, by definition, upsets the balance of safety, trust, and security. Illness exposes an individual to lack of safety, mistrust, and insecurity. It is important to assess how much an illness threatens safety, trust, and security. How an individual perceives threat to these basic needs determines how effective any form of interpersonal assistance will be.

The turtle who withdraws its head and legs into its protective shell when under assault is a useful image. The turtle has perceived a threat; its safety and security is imperiled and the environment is judged untrustworthy. Commonly we have used this image to understand the subtle defensive behaviors of human persons who seek protection in a variety of physical and psychological withdrawal behaviors.

AIDS is perceived by most infected persons to be a very threatening enemy. Not only does it destabilize the functioning of the body's immune system, but it also can negatively affect basic psychological functioning. What relevance does this have for pastoral care?

For an interpersonal relationship to be helpful, the person being helped needs to experience the helper and the environment as trustworthy, safe, and secure. In a pastoral relationship it takes time, skill, and patience to establish these foundational experiences.

David was very distressed. His deteriorating physical health and the recurrence of the PCP infection dictated his decision to move back to the east coast. Although he was receiving competent care in a major medical center in Connecticut where he was hospitalized, he did not feel as secure as he did at San Francisco General Hospital. He wondered whether the persons in charge of his care in Connecticut had as much knowledge about AIDS as did the staff in California.

He had always experienced difficulties in self-disclosure. He was circumspect in talking about his personal life, both with his family and with the professionals who cared for him. He did not offer information, and was guarded in how he answered direct questions. It appeared he had some perceived fears about how the information he communicated would be received and used.

It is important for a pastor to be sensitive to these issues. It will take time to gain David's trust. He has been away from institutional religious practice for a number of years of his adult life. During these years the Church has not been perceived as a welcoming place for him. He does not see the Church as a safe haven. It is not easy to change immediately those perceptions of the Church. People don't make transitions simply because they are seriously ill and are approached by a chaplain.

David may perceive the institutional Church as a further threat to his security. He may feel vulnerable to being rejected or condemned by the Church's judgments on him. He is not sure whether this priest is comfortable with a person with AIDS. He doesn't know whether the chaplain is tolerant and accepting of a gay man. He has no sense about this priest's abilities or inabilities to help him process the kinds of concerns he has on his mind. In sum, he is unsure.

All of these issues require assessment and response by the pastor. Only when a pastor understands David's basic needs can he begin to respond to them. David will need considerable reassurance if he is to be able to benefit from a pastor's counsel and ministry. It is inconceivable that he would have ever been able to respond affirmatively to the priest's invitation: "Make your confession and I'll give you the sacrament of the sick." The turtle would quickly withdraw its exposed members deep into its shell with such an approach to pastoral ministry.

Self-Esteem

There are many things that affect self-esteem. Some of the stresses we have already identified impact on self-esteem. A person's perceived inabilities to supply for his or her own basic physical and psychological needs can also weaken self-esteem. In our culture, a person's worth is often defined as a function of what he or she is able to do. Changes in self-esteem may be dramatic, but more often they are gradual, and sometimes imperceptible to others.

David was an accomplished individual. After completing college, he went to a prestigious west coast law school, was hired in a top firm, and his career flourished. He was a respected attorney in the corporate law offices in which he was employed. Since his earliest days, David had been independent. While maintaining contact with his family, he did not depend on them for support. Until his physical health began to decline after his initial bout with PCP, he had never required their assistance.

These few facts interpret David's vulnerability to weakened self-esteem. Mental health practitioners are alert to issues that weaken self-esteem and work to help individuals maintain and improve their self-esteem. Since mental outlook has a significant role either in improvement in health and functioning or in the progression of illness, this is something that demands attention.

A pastor's role in self-esteem maintenance or enhancement is also important. As noted before, the physical care of a person with AIDS is so demanding and time-consuming that there may be less time available to respond to psychosocial issues. Competent pastoral care can respond effectively to these needs. In order to do this, a pastor needs to make some assessments about how the diagnosis of AIDS is affecting the individual's self-esteem.

In David's situation, he was dubious about his ability to survive his second bout with Pneumocystis. He was not hopeful about returning to his job, his home, or his friends. He was uncomfortable thinking about his dependency on his brother and family. He was attributing responsibility for his illness to himself, blaming his lifestyle and previous choices for his present condition. He felt he had disappointed a number of people, most of all himself. The wish to die, though not verbalized, occupied his thoughts. He felt like a person alone on an island, with few resources and overwhelming challenges. All his former ambition, drive, self-confidence, and determination were gone. He was gradually assuming the passive role of victim. A few quick words of encouragement or some trivial cliche will not be an adequate antidote to the AIDS related problems of self-esteem with this person.

Strengths

In much of this chapter we have focused on a number of areas of needs of a person with AIDS. The discussion has necessarily uncovered areas of deficit that are related to the presence of a life-threatening illness. The point in this discussion has been to stress the importance of accurate assessment of these needs prior to any attempts to provide specific pastoral care to a person with AIDS.

Important also is an assessment of the patient's strengths. These can be important resources upon which to build. In the face of the many disabling aspects of AIDS, we may sometimes overlook the fact that a person has resources which are not necessarily weakened by the disease. Let's return to take a final look at David's case.

David's illness has not affected his thinking and reasoning. He is quite alert and attentive. This is an important resource to consider. From his days in high school, David has been a successful debater. He is a natural conversationalist, easy to engage in discussion. He is able to be persuaded as well as to influence another person's thinking. This characteristic of his personality remains functional in his illness and can be utilized in strategizing pastoral care.

A second area of strength in David's case is his basic coping mechanism. His characteristic independence has taught him how to solve many of his own life problems. He is not easily defeated. In his work, he persisted in difficult business negotiations long after some of the other attorneys in the firm would have aborted the process. He saw most things through until completion. To be able to engage this strength will be important not only in pastoral care, but in his continued will to live.

Finally, David is a fundamentally spiritual person. Although he abandoned the formal practices associated with the Roman Catholic faith, he nonetheless had an interior life. From his youth he internalized the essentials of his Christian heritage, maintaining a belief in God and a sense of his social obligations toward other persons. He was a consciously moral individual, and this sense of morality was evident in his personal and professional life. This strength will be important to call upon in the pastoral relationship.

6

Terminal Care of
Persons with AIDS

Throughout this book, we have described AIDS as a life-threatening illness. Many persons with AIDS, supported by a network of helpers including family, lovers, friends, health care professionals, volunteers, and clergy, marshal enormous inner resources in their struggles to cope with this disease. For a significant number of these persons, there comes a time in the course of the disease when AIDS is more properly described as a terminal illness. In this chapter we shall direct our attention to some issues involving the support and care of the terminally ill person with AIDS.

As we have seen, persons with AIDS depend on an extensive network of other individuals as they face multiple battles with this disease. We have noted how important it is that persons with AIDS retain maximum control over their lives as they face the vagaries of recurring and new infections. For this reason, it is imperative that those who offer to provide assistance assess accurately the needs and abilities of the person for whom they attempt to provide help. Becoming dependent upon others is a common experience of most persons who are seriously ill. As a person progresses closer to death, dependent relationships become more significant, and sometimes problematic.

Care-providers must learn to balance a dying person's need to retain autonomy and control over his or her life with the realistic requirements of providing physical care and emotional support. Pastoral ministry to a person dying of AIDS needs to consider this challenge to achieve balance.

The Pastor and the Terminally Ill Person

It is not an uncommon phenomenon that as persons move closer to death, they begin to limit the number of their interpersonal contacts. This natural tendency on the part of a dying person to restrict contact is difficult for those who provide care. It is painful for the persons in a support network who have provided varied forms of assistance during the long course of a person's illness to gradually be excluded from a dying person's interpersonal world. Some interpret the exclusion as ingratitude or rejection. In reality, the limitation of interpersonal contact is a normal psychological strategy which helps a dying person maintain limited control over his or her remaining life.

In their interactions with terminally ill persons, pastors may assume the legitimacy of their place in the life of the dying person. Because of their particular ministerial role and function, they may presume they have automatic entree into the life of the person and his or her family. This may be a false assumption. Not all dying persons desire or will accept the support of a pastor. Prior experiences with the pastor or religion, the personality and sensitivity of the particular minister, the stage in the dying process, and other variables affect a dying person's openness and receptivity to pastoral interventions.

Marilyn Krant, a thirty year old mother of three young children, died of AIDS. She contracted the disease as a result of surgery-related transfusions of contaminated blood which she received in 1982. During her heroic eighteen month struggle with the disease, her husband Todd was a constant support. With the assistance of a team of hospice professional staff and volunteers, Todd was able to provide home care for Marilyn during the terminal stage of her illness. Their minister, Rev. Vernon Clinton, pastor of United Methodist Church where they were members, was an important support to the family.

From the time of Marilyn's diagnosis, the Krants turned to Rev. Clinton for guidance and support. The pastor was immediately responsive to the family, and was with them throughout the long and difficult months of Marilyn's illness. In the final weeks of her life, Marilyn looked forward to Rev. Clinton's regular visits, to their conversations, and to the times in which they read Scripture and prayed. Although it was clear from her expressed needs and non-verbal behaviors that she preferred to limit the number of family, friends, and volunteers who were caring for her and assisting Todd, she never gave any indication that she wished to limit her contacts with Rev. Clinton. She often would ask Todd if the minister was coming on a particular day. Even when she was not feeling well, she was comforted when the minister would visit.

Rev. Clinton remained an important part of the Krants' support network, especially during the terminal stage of Marilyn's illness. The minister was always sensitive to his place in the family's life. He never came to their home without first calling and ascertaining whether his visit would be desirable. As Marilyn moved closer to her death, the minister was able to help her to talk about her dying. She seemed comforted by his willingness to participate with her in this way. One day when Rev. Clinton was with her, she asked Todd to sit with them as she discussed with the minister her desires for the memorial service after her death. Although this was a difficult experience for Todd, the minister was able to provide comfort to both of them as they planned for Marilyn's funeral.

Rev. Clinton was not with the Krants when Marilyn died, but he came to the home to be with the family soon after he received the news of her death. Todd expressed his gratitude to the minister for the support he had given to Marilyn and to the whole family during their long crisis with AIDS. Quoting the psalmist, Todd told Rev. Clinton that he had been "our rock and our refuge" during their eighteen month ordeal. Todd told him that of all the wonderful people who had helped him and Marilyn and the kids, he had been one of the most important.

In this case, the minister continued to maintain an important relationship to the dying person and her family. He was aware that his role, to a great extent, was determined by the dying person's needs and desires. He was willing to allow Marilyn to exercise control over the frequency and duration of their contacts, the topics they explored in their conversations, and the other individuals she wished to admit to their relationship. In the terminal stage of her life, the minister helped her talk about her dying, not only with her husband, but with her children, parents, and her only sister. It was clear that Rev. Clinton did not presume to have an important place in this family's crisis, but was willing to assume such a function and to modify it according to their changing needs. In this way, he was able to be a significant help to them during the entire course of Marilyn's illness and death.

However, not all attempts to offer pastoral assistance are welcomed. The following case highlights the problems some pastors encounter in ministering to persons with AIDS. Fr. Strickler received a call from the mother of a young man who was hospitalized with Pneumocystis. His condition was deteriorating rapidly, and the mother feared that he would die soon. This was his third hospitalization since his diagnosis nine months earlier. He returned home to be cared for by his aged parents. The mother was Roman Catholic; the father had not been religious. Rudy had been baptized and confirmed as a Catholic, but had not practiced his faith throughout his adult life.

Mrs. Miller was anxious about her son's declining health, and feared that he might die without receiving the sacraments of the Church. In her call to Fr. Strickler, she told him of Rudy's condition, and that she would very much appreciate it if the priest would visit her son in his hospital room. She told Fr. Strickler that Rudy had AIDS, "that terrible disease," hastening to add, "But Rudy's a good boy, Father, even though he's been involved with those homosexuals." Fr. Strickler assured her that he would arrange to visit Rudy.

When Fr. Strickler appeared at Rudy's room the next day, he found Rudy extremely weak. He was having great difficulty with his breathing, and required oxygen to ease his respirations. He was surprised to see the priest enter his room. They had never met before.

Rudy was minimally responsive to the priest's initial comments. He acknowledged that he understood his mother's call to the priest, but quietly said that he did not wish to talk with Fr. Strickler. The priest persisted in attempting to reach the dying man. As the priest continued speaking, Rudy became more and more agitated. Finally, Rudy said: "I don't believe in God, and I don't want to talk with you. If my mother needs your help, then help her. Please leave me alone."

The priest was startled by the patient's outburst. As Rudy completed his sentence he slumped back more deeply into his pillow and began to cough. He turned his head away from the priest as if to say, "Please leave now so that I will not have to look at you again." The priest retreated from the room, bewildered by the harsh rejection he had experienced. He was confused by Rudy's reaction, presuming that Mrs. Miller had discussed her request with her son prior to the priest's visit. He had assumed that his visit would have been appreciated, and that his ministry would have brought consolation not only to Mrs. Miller, but more importantly to her dying son. The flat rejection of his offer of pastoral support was upsetting to the priest. As he left the hospital, reflecting on his experience, he was angry, feeling that he had been manipulated. Returning to the rectory he called Mrs. Miller to report that he had attempted to visit her son, but that Rudy was unwilling to see him. The mother was discouraged by the communication, but thanked the priest for his efforts.

The experiences of Rev. Clinton and Fr. Strickler represent two different experiences of pastoral interventions with terminally ill persons with AIDS. They underscore the point that a dying person may or may not be receptive to the kinds of care a pastor may be willing and able to provide. However, a majority of dying persons, even those who may not have been actively religious prior to their illness, are responsive to appropriate offers of spiritual assistance by sensitive and non-judgmental pastors. Let us look at some of the specific issues pastors encounter in terminal care interventions.

AIDS and the Reawakening of Personal Spirituality

The confrontation with personal mortality can set in motion several dynamics. One of these involves the deepening or awakening of spirituality. In attempting to articulate what spirituality means in his book, *AIDS: The Spiritual Dilemma* (1987) John Fortunato writes:

By *spiritual* I allude to the journey of the soul—not to religion itself but to the drive in humankind that gives rise to religion in the first place. I have in mind the software on the computer of life, not its hardware; the program as it runs, not the data to be input or the machine that processes it or even the printout. By *spiritual* I am referring to that aura around all of our lives that gives what we do meaning, the human striving toward meaning, the search for a sense of belonging. (pp. 7–8)

Many individuals who are terminally ill, and who previously would not have considered themselves to have had a discernible spirituality, experience feelings which are properly spiritual. For some these feelings are comforting while for others they are confusing or disturbing. Pastors can be resourceful in helping persons make sense of these experiences. The following case describes the reawakening of these experiences.

Tad Gilford was a very successful neurologist who had married while he was in medical school. Coming to terms with his homosexuality, he divorced his wife after four years of marriage, entered into a relationship with a lover, and moved to the west coast to establish a new practice. Although his relationship with his lover was committed, he nonetheless had numerous casual sexual relationships with other men. During all of these years, he considered himself to be agnostic, although he had been raised and educated in the Roman Catholic Church. He had not practiced his religion since the end of his high school years. His lover was likewise a nominal Roman Catholic.

The summer before he was diagnosed with Kaposi's sarcoma, Dr. Gilford wrote a letter to a priest whom he had known while in college. During his undergraduate years he was actively questioning his faith and rebelling against the dogmatic positions of the Catholic Church. He frequently discussed these issues with a priest who had been his dormitory housemaster and who became his friend. The priest had officiated at his marriage to Karen, and had remained in occasional contact with him throughout the intervening years. The following is an excerpt from Tad's letter.

It's been an interesting summer for me. Work is as demanding as ever, and my practice continues to grow. Lee (his gay lover) and I separated more than eight months ago after five years together. It was a difficult, but necessary separation. We have both found the transition hard, but we are both so busy in our work that there isn't much time to dwell on the pain.

You may wonder why I am writing to you after so many months of silence, and so many years since we last saw each other. (I think the last time I saw you was just after my divorce from Karen, when I met Lee. That's almost six years ago.) Well, the simple reason for this letter is that recently I have been thinking about you a lot. I think it has to do with a spirituality which you felt within me at a time when I couldn't feel it myself. And now I'm feeling it more.

After Lee and I split up, I began to jog each morning. As you know, I was never much into athletics or exercise programs. Doctors can be notorious in not taking care of themselves! However, at my last physical, my internist advised that a modest exercise program might help to manage my slightly elevated blood pressure and some of the stresses I have been experiencing. Surprisingly, I have enjoyed running.

Well, running became the catalyst for doing some reflection. I've become aware of movements within me that, for lack of a better word, I describe as "spiritual." You are probably saying, "Well, Tad has finally come to terms with God." I don't know if I've come to terms with God, but I know something is coming alive within me.

When I was in college, we had many long debates about religion. On one occasion you told me, "Tad, you are fighting many battles within yourself and with the Church. Regardless of the ways in which you resolve these struggles, you have to recognize that there is a deeply spiritual core to your personality." I rejected that statement outright, confusing "spiritual" with being affiliated with the Catholic Church. When I concluded that I no longer believed in God, I likewise believed that I could not be spiritual.

Your words, you see, have stayed with me for almost thirteen years. This summer, during my spiritual reawakening, I have come to understand the meaning of your words.

*You must have seen something in me then that I could not
have seen. I don't know where all of this will take me, or
what it fully means, but I wanted to share this experience
with you. I know that God loves me. I walk a different path,
and at times feel at least temporarily abandoned. But
slowly, and more each few months, someone very good in me
is being nurtured.*

*I hope your life remains as full as I presume it is. I hope
you are well, and continue to grow. Something within you
glows. I hope this letter finds you at peace and leaves you
with happiness.*

In October of 1985, four months after he wrote this letter,
Tad noticed some lesions on his chest. Believing them to be
Kaposi's sarcoma lesions, he sought a consultation with a San
Francisco physician who had treated many KS patients. After
examining him and completing a biopsy, the diagnosis was confirmed. Tad qualified for an experimental program at UCLA and
immediately began treatment. He had a positive attitude toward
his illness, and though knowledgeable and realistic about his
survivability, he nonetheless realized that he could die within
the next couple of years.

In June of 1987 Tad Gilford died. During the months between his diagnosis and his death, he became a frequent corre-
spondent. His letters and telephone conversations with Father
Bradley were important to him. Although separated on the two
coasts, the geography did not seem to be a major obstacle to
their relationship. Tad seemed content that he had a person who
understood the spiritual developments taking place within him.
One of his early letters, soon after his diagnosis, expresses his
feelings:

*When I wrote to you last July about my spiritual re-
birth, I never thought that I would understand so soon the
"why" of the experience. AIDS and my likely death from it
has provided the key to its interpretation. If my spiritual
rebirth had occurred after my diagnosis with KS, I would
have been skeptical, figuring this was a panic reaction, a*

security blanket, a regression to my past. But God, it seems, was preparing me for this crisis.

My days have been very busy dealing with my physical needs. My physical and mental health are good. I have completed four weeks of beta interferon therapy. The first week I had to go to UCLA each day so that they could monitor temperature and blood pressure after the injections.

It was an interesting five days. Each day I would see different cancer patients, lots of them, young and old, with different kinds of cancer. There was a pregnant woman I saw twice, and several families with young children. I realized that I'm not the only person with a bad illness.

And everyone who works there has a quality of compassion that is impressive—from the receptionists to the lab technicians to the pharmacists to the doctors, and, most of all, the two nurses working with my doctors. It starts with a way of speaking, a quality in the voice that expresses a certain empathy. Then there is the ability to listen, one of life's greatest gifts.

Sometimes we would have half an hour between vital sign checks, and rather than doing paper work that eventually has to be done, either Judy or Suzy would sit with me and talk and listen. There is an oncology fellow, Steven Kirk, in his early thirties, maybe even younger, very bright, loves his work. I asked him how he can do this work. He smiled, and said that he doesn't approach his work with the same expectations that a neurologist has. He said that he helps people through a very difficult time in their lives. He said that he sees people in a very angry state when they first come in, and that often a lot of that anger is directed at him, but that as time passes and they go through the experience together something else builds. I was surprised and happy to have a doctor who is really in tune with what it is all about. He comes from a family of twelve children (Catholic, not Mormon), and his mother is a nurse. I felt as though a very good relationship was established that first week. . . .

The positive reinforcement I received at UCLA has helped me tremendously in formulating what amounts to a plan, a strategy, for dealing with this illness which combines physical, intellectual, emotional, and spiritual resources. I wish I could say that many other people with AIDS have received this same quality of care, but, unfortunately, that is not the case.

You probably know more horror stories than I do. In the past three weeks I have met two other men with Kaposi's sarcoma who have been told by physicians to do nothing about it. The medical rationale, if you can call it that, is that in the majority of cases, KS is a cosmetic illness whose principal complication is disfigurement if lesions begin to appear on the head and neck. This is true, but this rationale ignores the underlying killer virus which will inevitably lead to lethal infections. Thus, by telling the patient to go home and drink water (one of the men I met was told this by a reputable private physician in San Francisco), a very negative message is delivered.

Even the medically unsophisticated person knows that all people with AIDS die. By being told not to treat this condition, learned helplessness is encouraged, and the acquisition of subsequent adaptive learning is delayed or wiped out. Talk about depression. Talk about a perfect way to push gay people and IV drug users, two groups who already feel alienated from the system, away from good medical care, which does have certain options to offer. Worse yet, these people then end up in the hands of the charlatans who charge money to tell them to drink peroxide, or eat lentils, or spend half their income buying exotic vitamins and minerals, or holding crystals over the Kaposi's lesions. I am convinced that these problems have significantly contributed to the short survival of many AIDS patients.

Other than the KS lesions on my chest I haven't had any other symptoms. However, I've decided to withdraw from my medical practice, and have already spoken with my associates. I bought a grand piano and have begun to practice again. Although I lost much of my technique, I am amazed how much I still remember, and how quickly certain things come back. I'm very involved in the medical management of my illness, and have been in contact with the major people around the country who are involved in research and treatment. My medical background gives me access to people and information that others would not have. I believe that the process that I went through of investigating all options, and choosing the one that I believed was the best, has made all of this more comfortable. It makes the side-effects of the drugs easier to take, and, I think, physically less uncomfortable.

Even if this therapy does not work, I will feel satisfied that my choice was correct (interferon is said to produce remissions of KS in thirty to forty percent of patients). I am going after the visible cancer and the virus which I can visualize in my blood cells. My anger about my illness has started to be directed at the lesions themselves. I have various fantasies. Sometimes I fantasize about mutilating them, cutting them out with a crude knife. Or injecting them with a sclerosing solution. Or sitting under a radiation machine and cooking them. When I inject my interferon, I often fantasize about this solution sending my body's protecting cells to attack these lesions. Some of my thoughts are more gentle. I meditate on the healing powers that I know I possess, and try to direct them to melt the virus, and to make the skin lesions softly fade away.

My anticipation for the future is that I don't think I'm very frightened by the physical suffering. And I don't think I'm very frightened by the idea of my death. I feel a great strength growing within me. In the past few weeks, as I mentioned, I have met two men with a diagnosis like mine. I've been able to help them. In doing so, I could feel a talent God has given me being used to help my fellow man. In doing this, I could feel my own strength as it poured out to these men. I felt stronger, and yet at the same time I could feel my own pain more as I felt the pain of these men. But it was all very healthy.

If I am to be one of a new group who will be long-term survivors of this illness, it will be because of the best medical care, and the utilization of my strength and courage for myself and for others who are suffering. And, of course, the love and strength of my friends will also be part of it, and already has been, to the point where I know I'm O.K. And if it is my destiny to die from this illness, I'm beginning to understand what I have to do first. In all of this I feel God.

Apart from the medical issues, the most important of my current experiences is the spiritual movement within me. I am going to need your help now more than ever before to make sense out of all of this. One thing I realize is that you do understand what I'm talking about. Many of my friends with whom I have shared some of my "spiritual" experiences are puzzled and silent. It's an area where some of them have not walked. It was a lark that I wrote to you last summer after such a long silence. God must have been getting me ready for this major confrontation with life and its meaning.

I deeply appreciated your call last Tuesday, and your reassuring words, and your prayers. At least now I am able to accept your prayers. It was helpful to hear you say that you would continue to be with me throughout this crisis, and that you would be willing to fly out to visit if I needed you. Right now, I don't need that, but it was wonderful to hear you say those words. There is a good chance I will be in New York for Thanksgiving. Maybe I could arrange a detour and visit with you in person. Next time we talk on the phone, let me be the one to call you. The last call must have put you into the poor house. I think we talked almost two hours.

Writing this letter has felt wonderful. I know I am writing to someone who understands and cares. Thanks, Padre. I love you.

Tad's spiritual needs vacillated during the course of his terminal illness. He experienced the closeness and the distance of God. He felt divine love and forgiveness and was subjected to fears of God's abandonment and condemnation. He had times of intense consolation, and other moments of desolation. There were times when he was attracted to pray and read favorite passages in the Scriptures; at other times he had no attraction to any of these things and began to question again the authenticity of his spiritual experience. In each of these experiences, he needed the support and encouragement of his spiritual companion. As he approached his death, he acknowledged how important this relationship had been to him. In his words, "Nobody else could have reached so deeply into my soul and understood."

If the pastor is admitted into the support network of a terminally ill person with AIDS, he or she has an important contribution to make. Pastoral care is a healing ministry, even in the face of physical death. The pastor is frequently confronted with the challenge to support the healing of the human spirit, which AIDS, a person's lifestyle and relationships, and accumulated life experiences may have fractured. A dying person needs assistance as he or she strives to make sense out of life and to achieve a sense of wholeness and integration. Personal and communal prayer, scriptural meditation, practices of contemplation, and selective spiritual reading can all help the dying person to achieve this inner peace. However, the pastor must exercise restraint and good judgment as he or she helps the dying person to explore the spiritual dimensions of the terminal experience. It is unwise to attempt to force these experiences. The pastor must be discerning, respectful, and supportive of the initiatives of the dying person. One can suggest but not command, lead gently but not coerce. The prayer of Solomon (1 Kgs 3:5–12) could serve as a model for spiritual ministry to persons with AIDS:

> O Lord, my God, you have made me your servant . . . but I am a mere youth, not knowing how to act. I serve you in the midst of the people whom you have chosen, a people so vast that it cannot be numbered or counted. Give your servant, therefore, an understanding heart to judge your people and to distinguish right from wrong.

Working with Experiences of Isolation and Abandonment

Dying is essentially a solitary activity. Although a dying person may have the supportive presence of significant others, a dying person can often feel alone and isolated. The stigma associated with dying from AIDS, antipathy for individuals in high risk groups most affected by the disease, and abandonment by family, lovers, or friends may intensify the experience of isolation for a dying person. Finally, the Church may have been experienced as distant and rejecting.

Effective pastoral care is not necessarily an antidote to a

dying person's feelings of isolation and abandonment. However, it can make a significant contribution toward reconciliation of relationships and remediation of those issues which contribute to the negative feelings. Let us consider some practical ways in which feelings of isolation and abandonment can be addressed.

The first issue for the pastor is availability. In order to be helpful, one must be present. One of the commonly expressed concerns of many terminally ill persons is that people will leave them, and that they will be alone. Presence is of crucial importance. It is reassuring and comforting. Pastors need to realize how important it is that they be physically present. A dying person knows the competing demands made upon a pastor's time. He or she simply requires knowing when the pastor might return. It is not helpful to make promises about availability that are not realizable. It is important that promises to a dying person be kept; not to do so can have a psychologically destructive effect on the individual.

Secondly, the pastor needs to be practical in the goals he or she sets for his or her interventions. In some individual cases, dramatic reconciliations within families do take place; some individuals do have "deathbed conversions," and unresolved issues are settled. However, it is unreasonable to expect that each pastoral intervention with a dying person is going to be able to achieve all of these objectives. Goal setting in pastoral care is a collaborative activity. The dying person is an indispensable participant in reviewing what should or should not be attempted, what can or cannot be achieved. Active listening on the part of the pastor will help clarify what realistically can be expected.

And, finally, the pastor must be patient. Even though there is limited time to achieve modest goals in one's work with a terminally ill person, the process cannot be accelerated simply because the individual is dying. Many people die without completing their work. Quality of care, not quantity of goals achieved, is the priority in any pastoral initiative. Reconciliation of relationships and remediation of conflictual issues require calm persistence. They cannot be forced, even when there are major time constraints.

Denise and Larry had been married for nine years at the

time of Denise's diagnosis with AIDS-related lymphoma. She had undergone months of diagnostic evaluations before the AIDS diagnosis could be confirmed. She did not fit into any of the high-risk groups, and her sexual history was monogamous. Larry, on the other hand, had been involved in extramarital homosexual activity, although Denise had been unaware of this. Larry had great difficulty acknowledging this hidden aspect of his sexual life. He tested positive for the virus. It was reasonable to assume that he had infected his wife.

Both Denise and Larry had promising careers in commercial real estate. Although they looked forward someday to beginning a family, they had concentrated during the early years of their marriage in building their careers and increasing their financial base. Denise's illness and anticipated death quickly exploded those dreams. Denise felt as if she were drowning in a sea of conflictual feelings when Rev. Cheryl Rowe began to work with her. Rev. Rowe, a United Church of Christ minister and assistant chaplain at the community hospital in which Denise was being treated, was able to establish rapport and trust with her. Although neither Denise nor Larry was religiously active, both had been raised in conservative Protestant traditions.

Rev. Rowe encouraged Denise to express many of the feelings which were troubling her. She felt hate and love for Larry; she felt victimized, betrayed, and abandoned. Coming to know about Larry's homosexual behaviors, Denise felt somehow responsible. She mused about whether she was culpable because she did not adequately meet his sexual needs. She felt that her disease was punishment from God, because she and Larry had been distant from God, and almost exclusively focused on their own material prosperity.

Denise's parents and family were pained to learn about her terminal diagnosis, and were shocked and horrified by the implications of how she may have contracted the deadly virus. Their reactions to Larry were hostile and rejecting. Denise's father expressed his angry feelings to Larry in an ugly hospital confrontation. His language was loud and abusive, almost resulting in physical assault. He kept repeating the phrase, "That queer has killed my daughter." Hospital security had to be called to manage the conflict. As a result of that encounter, Denise felt caught in the middle of the battle, attempting to remain open both to Larry and to her own family. Rev. Rowe understood how the tensions Denise felt were contributing to her alienation.

Over the course of the final two months of Denise's life, Rev. Rowe became a significant person. The chaplain spent time each day with Denise, and met with Larry and his wife together. The chaplain also spoke with Denise's parents and other members of the family. She was able to help Denise sort through many of her conflictual feelings, and to use prayer and meditation to make peace with some of these discordant feelings. One of the most significant pastoral interventions was to help Larry seek pardon from his wife, and for Denise to express forgiveness to Larry. Rev. Rowe prepared each of them for this experience and facilitated the meeting in which this healing exchange took place. The process brought Larry and Denise closer together, and both were more peaceful as a result of the pastoral initiative. Rev. Rowe was less successful in her work with Denise's family, although they understood that their hostile attitudes toward Larry caused Denise added stress. They avoided Larry, and did not bring his name up in their conversations with Denise during her last days.

Rev. Rowe also worked with Denise and Larry to formulate her funeral plans. Together they selected readings and hymns for a simple memorial service. Denise asked Rev. Rowe to conduct the service in the small non-sectarian chapel within the hospital, and she agreed to do so. Denise asked Rev. Rowe to stay in contact with Larry after her death, because she felt he would need someone to talk with. Denise recognized that Larry was concerned about whether he would get sick with AIDS, and was preoccupied with the thought that no one would be there to take care of him. Recognizing how important this last wish was for Denise, Rev. Rowe assured her that she would remain in touch with him. Denise died peacefully, feeling that the Good Shepherd was beside her, leading her safely home. One important reason why she died with such reassurance and equanimity was that Cheryl Rowe did not abandon her.

The Search for Meaning in Death

How a terminally ill person approaches his or her own death is related to the meanings one has invested in life. This is more than a simple philosophical premise; it is important in understanding the psychological and spiritual aspects of the dying process. For example, an older person may see his or her life as God's plan, with each period of life having its own part to play in the unfolding of that plan. Death at the end of that process has its particular meaning as well. This view of life helps to explain the acceptance and the peacefulness with which many older persons face death.

Some people find meaning and purpose in their family relationships, in their friendships, in the works in which they are engaged. Some others may discover life's meaning in personal goals to be achieved. For example, a person may find meaning in life by conquering Mount Everest in the Himalaya Mountains of Tibet. Or another may find meaning in completing a degree program. While I was in graduate school there was a sixty year old man completing a doctoral program in psychology. When asked by his fellow students why he was putting himself through the rigors of a demanding study program, he said, "I want to have my name chiseled on my tombstone with the letters, 'Ph.D.' " He found meaning in life in that accomplishment. Still others may discover meaning by dedicating their lives to a specific purpose. For example, a woman could dedicate herself to a religious community and spend her life caring for the materially poor. Or a man could commit himself to a lifetime crusade to protect wildlife. The point of this discussion is to emphasize that death is linked inextricably to the meanings (or lack of meaning) that we find in living.

Many persons who are dying of AIDS are young. The relationships and experiences, the investments and the commitments which carry personal meaning may yet have to be accomplished. A diagnosis of AIDS and the prospect of an early death may challenge the meaning one can find in dying. It is reasonable to expect that those who have led the lives they desired will sense completion as they look forward to death. If this is generally true, then it is logical to assume that for those who have not lived as they had wished, their approach to death will be more problematic. AIDS and death significantly interrupt the possibilities of altering the life course one had been pursuing, or accomplishing what was left undone.

Pastors will necessarily be faced with questions involving meaning. Some of the questions terminally ill individuals frame are rhetorical, expressing concerns, fears or doubts, rather than seeking responses. Other questions are genuine searches for understanding, struggles to make sense out of personal experiences, disease, or dying. In each of these questions, pastors need to determine what it is that is being said, and how best to appropriately answer the person.

Jim was a forty-one year old college English professor. He taught in a small, prestigious private liberal arts college in New England. Raised in a family of professional educators, he went to private schools, an ivy league college and graduate school. In his field of English literature, he was a competent and popular teacher. His publication record was modest, but enough to earn him tenure at his institution. Jim lived alone, although he had been in two short-term relationships during the past dozen years since he entered the teaching profession.

Raised in a devout Anglo-Catholic home, Jim had remained involved in religious practice, serving as a member of the vestry of his St. Stephen's Episcopal Church. Jim was an active member of the parish, and respected by the clergy and parishioners. Few in the community knew of Jim's homosexuality, although some may have suspected it. Jim did not lead an overtly gay life, and was not actively involved in a gay network of friends. His sexual involvements tended to be anonymous. It was therefore a surprise to many when it was rumored that Jim had contracted AIDS.

Jim's health declined rapidly from the time of his initial diagnosis with Pneumocystis. He developed several other infections, which proved difficult to treat effectively. The rector of Saint Stephen's, Rev. David Massey, expressed his support for Jim from the first hours of his hospitalization. Jim felt more comfortable in sharing the secret aspects of his past life with Father Massey than he did with members of his family or other friends. There was not only a pastoral relationship, but a genuine friendship that existed between the two men. Father Massey became an important member of the care team during Jim's final illness.

As Jim told Father Massey the story of his life, the priest was surprised how little meaning was invested in Jim's professional accomplishments. Jim considered himself to be an average teacher and scholar; he was unenthusiastic about his work in the college, and did not consider many of his colleagues to be more than acquaintances. They were clearly not his friends. He regretted that he had not been able to come to terms with his homosexuality in a more acceptable way, and was disappointed that he had been unable to form a committed relationship with another individual. In describing his promiscuous lifestyle, he felt certain that he had contracted the disease through one or more of these anonymous encounters. There was a sense that he was ready to accept responsibility for getting infected with the AIDS virus because of his risky sexual history.

There were numerous things that Jim wished he had done differently with his life. He acknowledged that he entered the academic profession because of family pressures. He was never happy in that setting, even though he was judged to be successful. He wished that he had pursued an interest in broadcast journalism. Another regret was that he had not made peace with his sexual orientation earlier in his life, and perhaps been able to avoid the promiscuous ways in which he satisfied his sexual needs. The only area in which he found meaning was his relationship within the Church. Father Massey picked up on this and, with Jim's permission, helped to organize members of the parish to visit with Jim and assist him in the final months of his life.

Death was something that Jim feared. His fears were not linked to concern about the afterlife or God's judgment, but rather were related to things he would not be able to accomplish in his life, things to which he had attached hidden meanings. It was to some of these things that Father Massey responded, helping Jim to let go. In the area of his life where he found significant meaning—in his religion and Church associations—the priest was able to help him to consolidate those important experiences and bring them to bear on his process of dying. The

Church membership generally was responsive, and Jim derived considerable consolation from this form of pastoral care.

Making Peace with the Past

Dying has its unique way of calling in the outstanding debts from the past. Some have referred to this phenomenon as completing "unfinished business." This can involve dealing with interpersonal conflicts in familial relationships or friendships. It may entail working through difficulties that have contributed to alienation from God and the Church. It may be making peace with aspects of one's lifestyle and choices. In assisting a dying person to complete the "unfinished business," helpers must exercise great control by not imposing their own personal agenda upon the person who is making important choices.

As persons move closer to death, the hierarchy of personal values may shift, with some people and issues becoming more important than others. Clergy should not assume that religious issues or their own positions as pastors retain a place of importance in the dying person's life. Frequently dying persons do want the support and assistance of a clergyperson, but pastors need to be sensitive to the times when their presence becomes an additional burden to the dying person. Likewise, it is not uncommon that a dying person begins to disengage from relationships as he or she progresses toward death. This process, which is physical as well as psychological, may begin to selectively exclude people from contact. Pastors are not exempt from this selection process, and should not assume a place in the narrowing inner circle of contacts based on their roles as pastors. As long as a dying person signals or expresses a desire for a pastor's support, there are good opportunities to help the individual complete "unfinished business."

Because of the nature of pastoral ministry to persons who are terminally ill, pastors ordinarily encounter issues of "unfinished business." We should not underestimate the importance that dying persons place on these issues and concerns. A good deal of a person's remaining affective energy may be invested in these concerns. As noted before, we have emphasized the importance of helping sick and dying persons remain in control of their lives. They identify their own agenda, and determine when and under what circumstances they choose to address issues of concern.

It may be useful for the pastor to ask a dying person questions that might prove beneficial in facilitating resolution of some "unfinished business." However, questions should never be put in such a way that they suggest what a person should do or force compliance. "Are there some things that you might wish to discuss with me today? Things that are bothering you, things you have on your mind?" Some people readily respond to this line of questioning, outlining an agenda of things they want to complete. Others may respond positively, adding that today is not the right time to do this. Others may not be ready at all, and reply that everything is O.K. today. In these latter cases, it may be helpful to respond with an additional question: "Would it be O.K. to raise the same questions with you at another time, perhaps when you might be more ready to talk?" This method of questioning extends the courtesy of control to the dying person, respecting his or her right to identify and work through unfinished issues, allowing him or her to manage what is attempted and on which schedule.

Steven had recently celebrated his thirty-fourth birthday as he entered the terminal stages of his year and a half battle with AIDS. Raised in a large and supportive Irish Catholic family, he had been assisted throughout his illness by members of his family. He had two prior hospitalizations and each time had been able to return to his own apartment. His younger sister, Kathleen, a registered nurse, became the family's liaison, her brother's principal care-partner, and the coordinator of his support network.

For more than forty-five years, the O'Keefe family had been parishioners at St. Elizabeth's parish. The parents moved into their home two years after their marriage and there raised their seven children. The parish was an important center of their lives. All of the children attended the parish elementary school. Helen and Joe O'Keefe were active parishioners. Over the years they became close to many of the priests who had served the parish. Their home was an open and welcoming place.

When they learned of Steven's homosexual lifestyle at the time of his diagnosis with AIDS, they were upset and confused.

Despite the fact that they disapproved of homosexuality, they did not reject their son. When Steven was first hospitalized with AIDS, the O'Keefes called Father Nichols who responded to their request. He had been a young priest in St. Elizabeth's when Steven was a boy. Father Nichols, now pastor of another parish community, had been the director of the parish youth group in which Steven participated. They had remained close through the years.

Throughout the course of Steven's illness, Father Nichols continued to visit him. As he drew closer to death, Steven seemed to draw great comfort from his conversations with his priest friend. Kathleen commented that of all the people who visited Steven, Father Nichols seemed to be the one who most bolstered her brother's spirits.

Father Nichols was a direct person. His directness was helpful to Steven. As they talked about Steven's prior relationships, the priest learned that Steven had lived with another man for almost two years. They had a difficult parting. Father Nichols asked Steven if Jeremy had been in to visit. Steven replied that he had not. It was clear that Steven wished to see Jeremy and to attempt to reconcile the differences that contributed to their stormy separation four years ago. Steven had not spoken about this to Kathleen, or to any other family members, yet Father Nichols was astute enough to realize that this was an important part of Steven's "unfinished business."

With Steven's permission and assistance, Father Nichols was able to contact Jeremy by telephone, talk with him about Steven's deteriorating health and proximate death, and invite him to visit. The priest met with Jeremy prior to his visit with Steven. The encounter between Steven and Jeremy, though difficult for both men, was productive. After the visit, Father Nichols observed a significant change in Steven's behavior. He appeared more peaceful and more resigned. He thanked Father Nichols for contacting Jeremy, and for the understanding and support he felt. It was as if a major burden had been lifted from his shoulders. After Steven's death, Jeremy visited Father Nichols on two occasions to pursue his own grief work. Jeremy likewise was grateful that Father Nichols had recognized Steven's need for reconciliation and had been instrumental in helping it to take place before Steven died.

Unresolved Issues with the Church

For some dying persons alienated for a long time from the practice of religion, the approach of death may trigger a need for reconciliation. Some persons dying of AIDS may experience intense feelings of alienation, not only from former religious practice, but from society as well. This compounds the difficulties that pastors may encounter as they attempt to respond to these particular needs. Associated in the experience of some individuals with AIDS is the perception that they have been rejected by the Church. Some public religious figures have suggested that AIDS is a God-sent plague, his revenge on persons who have chosen to live perverted and irresponsible lifestyles. This position has been countered by other Church leaders who recognize the need for a more sympathetic and accepting approach to persons affected by the AIDS pandemic.

On April 8, 1987, the bishops of the California Catholic Conference published a pastoral letter on AIDS in which they attempted to quiet fears about the disease, to reflect upon the pandemic within the beliefs and traditions of Roman Catholicism, and to suggest ways of reaching out to care for and support persons with AIDS and their families. They affirmed that "as disciples of Jesus, we bear a special responsibility to care for the sick, to show them they are loved and to assure that they are treated with dignity and respect." The bishops recalled the ministry of Jesus who engaged in "an immediate, direct, hands-on ministry of healing" whenever he encountered a person who was sick or dying.

The bishops made specific reference to members of the homosexual community who are affected by the disease in significant numbers, "some of whom have been separated from the Church and its spiritual life." Responding to this fact, the bishops stated: "We regret this distance, and long to heal their wounds by offering our support and fellowship." They encouraged special preparation for all persons engaged in ministry to gay men or lesbian women which will make these ministers "more sensitive to the needs of this group."

The importance of providing non-judgmental and sensitive assistance to persons who are ill and dying of AIDS is a central concern of the California bishops' letter. The Church leaders acknowledged that as many other epidemics have done in the past, "the AIDS phenomenon provides a focus for the projection of fears and prejudices against infected persons and those in already marginated high-risk groups." Working against biases and prejudices, the bishops concluded: "People with AIDS/ARC remind us that they are not distant unfamiliar victims to be pitied or shunned, but persons who deserve to remain within our communal consciousness and to be embraced with unconditional love."

Earlier in this book we made reference to the death of Father Michael Peterson, a priest-psychiatrist and former director of Saint Luke Institute in Suitland, Maryland. Father Peterson died of AIDS in April of 1987. Writing to bishops and fellow priests before his death, Peterson said: "I hope that in my own struggle with this disease, in finally acknowledging that I have this lethal syndrome, there might be some measure of compassion, understanding, and healing for me and for others with it— especially those who face this disease alone and in fear." His bishop, Archbishop James Hickey of Washington, D.C., commented in response: "His tragic death is a reminder to each of us of the personal and human dimensions of this growing epidemic. Those suffering from AIDS are our brothers and sisters deserving our care, respect, and understanding. Father Michael's death challenges us to reach out to those with AIDS with renewed conviction and sharing."

These insightful and direct initiatives by Church leaders recognize the special needs of persons dying of AIDS, particularly those whose lifestyles may have contributed to their alienation from the Church. These problems are compounded when the person dying is black or hispanic. In the United States, persons of color make up more than twelve percent of the population, but account for twenty-five percent of all AIDS cases. Blacks and hispanics are at least twice as likely as whites to have AIDS. And among children with AIDS, a large number of whom become infected through prenatal maternal transmission, more than eighty percent of these are black or hispanic.

Charlie Wall was diagnosed with AIDS more than eight months ago. When his family and friends learned of his diagnosis, many of them abandoned him. He turned to the Church, AME Zion Church, for support. Speaking to his minister he commented that he wasn't afraid to die of AIDS, but that he didn't want to die alone. Charlie confessed to his minister that he knew the Church's views on homosexuality, and how hostile some black congregations can be to people known to be gay. Charlie told Rev. Washington, his pastor, that he hoped the Church would not abandon him because he was a gay black man.

Earlier on in the evolution of the AIDS pandemic, it was suspected that among whites in the United States, AIDS was spread principally by homosexual behaviors, while among blacks and hispanics the principal route of transmission was through intravenous drug use. These assumptions are not true. Statistics support the assertion that the higher proportion of AIDS cases in the black and hispanic populations are attributable to homosexual and bisexual behavior than to intravenous drug use.

This is not welcome news, particularly to those whose ministries to these minority populations have had to contend with the problems of racism, ethnic prejudice, and poverty. When associated with homosexuality, cases of AIDS in the black and hispanic communities add another level of discrimination. Contrasted with white gay men, black and hispanic men are often reluctant to admit to their homosexual behavior; although sexually active, many do not consider themselves to be "gay." When questioned about their sexual histories, a number of black and hispanic men create drug use histories rather than acknowledge homosexual activities. Many of the men involved in situations of male-to-male transmission are also sexually involved with women. Among black and hispanic men, homosexuality is a major taboo, which explains why there is extensive denial in these racial and ethnic populations.

Pastors serving blacks and hispanics with AIDS have special challenges. In these communities, the churches play important leadership roles, not only in social, religious and political spheres, but also in education. The predominantly conservative theological traditions of the majority of black and hispanic churches, their strong and articulate positions on sexuality, and their general opposition to homosexuality make ministry to persons with AIDS problematic.

Black and hispanic pastors are also concerned about the ways in which their respective congregations will respond to a more open and tolerant attitude toward members who become infected with the virus, develop AIDS, and die. These denominational churches tend to be small and numerous. Pastors are cautious not to alienate their communities which could threaten the particular church's survival. Already economically depressed with aging congregants, a number of the churches in black and hispanic communities do not see AIDS as a major problem they face. As a result, persons of color who contract AIDS and who face death may do so without effective support from the Church.

Sheila, a twenty-eight year old black woman, was diagnosed with AIDS. She was a single mother of two children, the youngest of which was born with AIDS. Sheila had been involved in intravenous drug use and prostitution. Although raised in a fundamentalist Southern Baptist family, Sheila had not been a practicing member of the Church. Her widowed mother, Corrine Samuels, with whom she lived, was a devout parishioner of Mt. Hope Baptist Church, sang in the church choir, and was devoted to the pastor, Rev. Clyde Brown. Mrs. Samuels had confided to Rev. Brown that Sheila and Jason were both diagnosed with AIDS.

Reverend Brown visited Sheila and attempted to be supportive to her. Sheila was uncomfortable with the minister's visits. She did not feel that he understood or respected her. His approach to her felt condemnatory of her lifestyle, implying that she was responsible for her predicament. His comments made her feel that Jason was conceived in sin, and that God was punishing her. Reverend Brown often quoted passages about repentance and forgiveness from the Bible. He seemed uncomfortable being with her, knowing that she had AIDS. He avoided mention of the fact that she had AIDS, that she was dying, or that her young baby was also seriously ill. Brown seemed intent on getting Sheila to repent of her sins and turn to Jesus.

Through these visits with Rev. Brown, Sheila became more depressed. Her mother frequently echoed many of the things Rev. Brown had said.

In the following months as Sheila grew weaker and closer to death, the Church became more remote to her. Her greatest comfort came from the nurses who cared for her in the hospital. They helped her to talk about her concerns for her older son whom her mother would raise. During her own extended illness, Jason died. The nurses and other hospital staff helped her to arrange for the burial of his body, to talk with Jimmy and to begin to prepare him for the death of his mother, and to help Mrs. Samuels to be of greater support to her dying daughter. In all of this, Rev. Brown became only a spectre to Sheila, a distant figure whose voice and message was more disturbing than comforting. Rev. Brown seemed incapable of ministering to the special needs of this family, although Mrs. Samuels continued to feel that the minister was a great help to her personally.

Dying with Dignity

Death from AIDS can be a horrendous experience. The disease in its many related expressions robs body and spirit of life. The provision of physical and emotional care depletes the resources of family and medical support staff. Assisting the person with AIDS to die with dignity, when faced with the other realities of this disease, represents a significant challenge.

In *The Screaming Room*, Barbara Peabody provides many insights into the problems of helping someone with AIDS to die in a dignified manner. The following passage is excerpted from her journal entries for November 7, four days before Peter's death.

> *Peter's lips move. I can't hear anything. He hasn't enough strength to blow breath through his words, to make them audible.*
> *"What is it, Peter?"*
> *He tries again. Nothing.*
> *"Peter, I can't tell what you're saying. It's all right, Peter." I wish I could read lips. I smooth his hair back on the*

painless side, raging at my helplessness. . . . *He is so thin,*
his face gaunt under the black beard. His unseeing eyes are
slightly open. The right eyeball shows whitely; only the left
pupil can be seen. His lips move. We try to understand his
voiceless words. Damn. Now when he needs to speak, he
can't. Not even my last dim hope is answered. . . .

    Everything is happening so fast. I feel helpless, con-
fused, dazed. I can't keep up. I wanted more time. Peter
wanted more time. I thought it would be slower, a few weeks.
Now it's down to days. The bucket is empty, the last drop
falling out and I can't catch it in my hands, scoop it back like
I could before. . . . *(pp. 238–239)*

Barbara Peabody, and many other parents, family, lovers, and friends of persons dying of AIDS, dedicate their energies to helping their loved ones find significance and dignity in the last phases of their living. In addition to providing essential medical and nursing support to insure maximum comfort and minimal pain, care-givers' efforts are directed to the emotional and spiritual needs of the dying person.

When we talk about a person with AIDS dying with dignity, we mean that every effort is made to insure that the individual's rights are safeguarded. Everyone admitted into the inner circle of contact with the dying person should be attuned to these issues. As noted before, as long as a dying person is conscious, he or she needs to retain control over decisions affecting care. But dying with dignity involves more than control in decision-making. A dying person needs to continue honest and meaningful relationships with important persons, needs to experience direct and affirming communication, needs to find meaning and purpose in the final stage of living, needs to be engaged in purposeful activities.

Pastoral care of terminally ill persons with AIDS must complement these essential goals of dignified dying. How one approaches a dying person, the effective communication of acceptance and respect for the person, and the commitment to support the person through the transition from life to death can contribute to the dying person's feelings of dignity. In working with gay men who are dying, pastors need to be accepting of relationships which continue to have significance and meaning to the dying person. Some pastors have experienced discomfort in witnessing demonstrations of physical affection between a dying person and his lover and friends. Approval of behavior and acceptance of those behaviors are distinct issues. Pastors do not have to approve of behavior in order to be accepting of another person's needs and choices.

By their acceptance, pastors assist dying persons to reduce remaining conflicts and tensions that might exist in their network of significant persons. With pastoral support and encouragement, dying persons may be able to resolve adequately interpersonal difficulties. Such resolution brings a deep experience of peace and completion, helping a person to die with dignity.

Finally, effective pastoral interventions can bring the consoling reassurance of God's presence and acceptance. Divine love is mediated through human contact. The focus of a pastor's prayers can help a person to accept the forgiveness and love of God. It can help the person, in the final moments of life, to let go, to surrender. A pastor's support can help a person to experience that the battle is over, the war has been fought. In this way the person of the pastor can be instrumental in assisting the dying person to bring a dignified closure to the final stage of living.

During the final weeks of his life, Father Mansell became very close to Lee. Lee, aged twenty-nine, had been living in a relationship with Rich. Throughout the fourteen months of his battle with Pneumocystis and other AIDS-related illnesses, Lee had the continual support of Rich. Lee's family had known of his homosexuality for many years, and had accepted it. They likewise had grown to love and respect Rich.

When it became necessary to care for Lee at home, they together decided that the best option would be for Lee to return to his parents' home. Rich and Lee had lived and worked in New York City. On weekends, Rich would stay with the Beckers in their home in Connecticut. They provided an additional bed in the room in which Lee was staying so that Lee and Rich could be together. The family included Rich in all of the decisions concerning Lee's care. This made Lee very happy. He looked forward to Rich's weekly visits. Rich was extremely faithful in calling and visiting. In the final months of Lee's life, he missed only one weekend, when he had a heavy cough and flu. He did not want to expose Lee to further infection.

Father Mansell was the parish priest in the Beckers' parish. He was new to the parish and had not met Lee prior to the terminal stage of Lee's illness which necessitated home care with his parents. Although initially uncomfortable working with a person who was gay and was seriously ill with AIDS, Father Mansell quickly adjusted and was able to establish a good relationship with Lee. While he was able, Lee had long and animated discussions with Father Mansell about a variety of topics. Father Mansell met Rich and had some helpful conversations with him and with Lee.

When Lee's pneumonia recurred and he was readmitted to the hospital, Father Mansell visited him daily. The family, as well as Rich, grew more dependent upon Father Mansell as Lee's condition worsened and death became a more inevitable outcome. Father Mansell had the ability to comfort Lee, Rich, and all the family. He spoke affirmingly of the love that bound them together; his prayers asked God for the grace of acceptance and resignation. Three days before Lee died, Father Mansell celebrated the Eucharist in Lee's hospital room, and all of the immediate family and Rich were present. Lee had asked to receive the sacrament of anointing during the celebration of the Mass, and Father Mansell anointed him with great sensitivity and compassion. After Lee's death, the family has many times recalled this special celebration. Rich said of Father Mansell, "I never thought a priest could be as loving as Father Mansell has been to us. He helped Lee and me to face the worst time in our lives with hope and love. And he has continued to stay in contact with me since Lee died. It has changed my opinion of the Catholic Church."

7

Ministering to Families of Persons with AIDS

Each person with AIDS is someone's son or daughter, someone's brother or sister, someone's parent, spouse, friend, or lover. AIDS is a family syndrome. It has its impact not only on the person whose body is infected with the deadly virus, but on each other person with whom he or she shares important relationships. BettyClare Moffatt in her monograph, *When Someone You Love Has AIDS* (1986), states it well:

> For every person who contracts AIDS, the entire family circle carries the consequences of that person's disease with them and carries, as well, the consequences of that AIDS person's decision to live hopefully or die despairingly. For every lover and every friend, for coworkers and health professionals, the AIDS person (not victim!) stands as a mirror for all our fears about disease, about death, about pain, about loss. Each one of us is confronted daily by our own deepest fears, our own personal response to life and death, our own choices to run away or to stay and love. In this connection the AIDS person serves as a metaphor for all our deepest fears about the disease and death (as well as our guilt over sex), and serves us well, in love, together with the one who confronts and triumphs over a tragic diagnosis. (p. 7)

In any crisis, the person who is afflicted draws the principal attention. In the AIDS crisis, the physical and emotional needs

135

of persons with AIDS command the considerable knowledge and attention of a competent team of care-providers. When we refer to the "family" of persons with AIDS, we include not only spouse, parents, children or siblings, but also friends and lovers who share important places in the afflicted person's life and care. Often enough, there is little time or attention available to address the special needs of family members. In this chapter we shall direct our focus to some of these needs and explore opportunities for effective response by individuals engaged in pastoral care.

The Stress of Learning About
an AIDS Diagnosis

A person with AIDS and his or her family share one thing in common: their lives are never the same once a diagnosis of AIDS is confirmed. A person with AIDS wakes up and retires each day, confronted with the realities of the disease; involved family members face the same daily prospect. A life-threatening illness modifies the values and perspectives of both the afflicted person and those individuals in his or her life who are most closely related to him or her.

Barbara Peabody recalls the morning—December 4, 1983— when her ex-husband, a physician, called to tell her that their son, Peter, was hospitalized in New York, having been diagnosed with AIDS. Excerpts from her journal capture her emotions:

> "Oh, my God, no-o-o!" My cry pierces the quiet, San Diego morning. I am cold, shaking uncontrollably. I clutch the blankets around me. . . . I can't speak. . . . I hang up and stare into space, my body still shaking. I am cold, frightened.
> I try to remember what I've read about AIDS. Dammit— what did that article say, where did I see it? Why didn't I pay more attention? After all, Peter is homosexual, and I know it affects homosexuals. . . .
> It can't be true. Peter is only 28, still trying to put his life together. It's not fair.
> Now I must speak to Peter.

The line crackles, hums. 3,000 miles disappear.
"Hello?" Peter's voice, weak, shadowy.
"Hi, Peter. It's Mom."
"Well, hi!"—as if it's an ordinary Sunday call. "How'd you know I was here?" I can barely hear his voice.
"Dad told me. He called this morning. How are you feeling?"
"Pretty good, I guess."
What else can he answer: "Terrible, I might die"? Small talk, but words are unimportant. We don't mention AIDS. He's alive, he's talking to me.
"I love you," I say in closing.
"I love you, too," he answers, his voice soft. We haven't said that to each other since he was a little boy.
I hang up the phone and cry. (The Screaming Room, pp. 1–4)

Learning about a loved one's diagnosis with AIDS is inherently stressful. This knowledge can catalyze a number of physical and emotional reactions, many of which are normal stress responses. Some of these include headaches, inability to sleep, stomach upset, loss of appetite, panting, sighing, or sporadic crying. The most common emotional reaction is depression. Family members feel numb, tense, experience difficulties in concentrating on tasks, and are unable either to work or to stop working. If family members do not pay attention to these signs of stress, then their own health may be compromised. A family member who wishes to help a loved one with AIDS must learn to manage and control these manifestations of stress.

Darlene and Daryl had a difficult marriage. For three years, Daryl had been serving a ten year sentence for a felony charge on which he was convicted. Recently paroled, they resumed their life together. Darlene had been sexually active with other partners during Daryl's incarceration, and Daryl had had some homosexual encounters while in prison. Darlene became pregnant soon after Daryl's release from prison. The baby, Samantha, was born with the AIDS virus, and at age six months developed the disease.

Both parents were upset, suspecting that the other spouse's sexual lifestyle was responsible for the baby's illness. Their relationship was not strong, and the crisis of an AIDS diagnosis, superimposed on the ordinary stresses of parenthood, was crushing.

The Baptist chaplain whom Daryl had met during his confinement in the State Correctional Institution learned of the Robinsons' crisis through Daryl's probation officer. He made immediate contact with the family and arranged to visit them in their apartment.

Rev. Johnson found the couple in a heightened emotional state. Samantha's development was retarded, and her general health was precarious. During the first two months of her life she had a bacterial infection, followed by a fungal infection. At the time of the minister's visit, Samantha had been hospitalized with a form of meningitis, and the prospects for her survival were not hopeful.

The Robinsons were grateful for the minister's visit. Their families had not been very helpful to the young couple. Fearful of becoming infected themselves, family members avoided Darlene and Daryl. Rev. Johnson was insightful and direct. He encouraged the couple to express their feelings. Their feelings included anger and blame, guilt and remorse, estrangement and fear. They were apprehensive about their own lives and future, whether they would get AIDS, since both of them tested positive for HIV. Rev. Johnson's presence and evident support helped Daryl and Darlene ventilate their feelings. Johnson listened and responded to their feelings and their questions.

For his part, the minister addressed those issues that he could begin to process with the couple. He spoke with them about God's care for them, not his wrath or punishment. He encouraged them to forgive each other, and to let go of their mutual feelings of blame and guilt. He helped them to see that Samantha needed her parents' love at this critical time in her life, and that this time would be important for the parents as well.

Before leaving them that evening, Rev. Johnson prayed with the couple for many of the things that had been topics of the discussion. He counseled them to participate in a group for family members of persons with AIDS. Knowing it would be difficult for them to make contact and enter the group, he asked if he could accompany them to the first meeting. They agreed and participated. Although they did not remain in the group for a long time, they did benefit somewhat from the experience, particularly during the weeks before Samantha's death. Johnson remained in contact with Daryl and Darlene, and officiated at a memorial service for Samantha which both Daryl and Darlene found to be comforting.

Another familial crisis surrounding a diagnosis of AIDS is the issue of a member's sexual orientation and practice. Although AIDS makes no distinction with respect to a person's age, gender, or sexual preference, a large percentage of cases in the United States is found among gay and bisexual men. The infection statistics have given rise to a popular understanding of AIDS as a "gay disease." This is factually not true, although common perceptions are not always based on factual evidence. For many families, the news that a relative has been diagnosed with AIDS raises latent questions about sexuality. Some spouses, parents, children, and siblings question the validity of the diagnosis, asserting that it could not be so because their husband, son, father, or brother isn't homosexual.

While many younger persons do share the fact of their sexual orientation with parents, siblings, and friends, for others this information remains secret. In the latter cases, the withholding of communication may be evidence of deeper problems of closeness or trust within family systems, or it may simply be that an individual judges that family members would be unable to handle well the disclosure. For whatever reasons, for some families the burden of learning that a member has AIDS is compounded by the realization that the same person is also gay.

Herbert Moore was a sixty-four year old successful business executive, married to his wife, Stephanie, for thirty-seven years. The Moores had three married children and seven grandchildren. For most of his adult life, Herbert had been involved in anonymous homosexual activities. Although his wife had some suspicions, she never openly confronted him about her concerns, nor did he share this information with her.

In response to his perceptions of declining energy and vulnerability to colds, Herbert was anonymously tested for HIV. Not only were his results positive, but his T-4 cells were alarmingly low. At his doctor's suggestion Herbert began a protocol of AZT medication. AZT is a drug which has shown promising results in controlling the AIDS virus.

With the knowledge of his positive test results and the beginning of his AZT medication program, Herbert decided to tell Stephanie. She was saddened to learn simultaneously of his bisexual activities and his HIV status. Nonetheless, she expressed her love and commitment to him. Together they began to consider how they would share the essential information with their children. At first they were reluctant to do so, but soon afterward they decided that it was important that their children be informed.

Families react to this dual communication with a variety of emotional responses. With respect to the news about the diagnosis of AIDS, most are stunned and fearful, unwilling to accept the full reality of the news. Many are shocked and numb, unable to believe that what they knew happened to other people's children was now happening to theirs. Learning about an adult child, parent, or spouse's homosexuality precipitates an even broader repertory of emotional responses.

Spouses, parents, children, siblings, and friends may be resentful and angry that they were not told the information earlier. They may be embarrassed by the news, concerned about how this information will be understood, interpreted, and accepted by other relatives and friends. They may feel betrayed, as though a person's homosexual orientation taints the family's image or reputation. Some family members become enraged, as if a gay brother's sexuality is a personal affront to the family's life. They may be hurt by the news, feeling guilty that they may have played some significant role in why a family member is gay.

With these confusing thoughts and heightened emotions family members often seek a trustworthy friend or a rabbi, minister, or priest. In doing so, they demonstrate a need to sort out the various levels of their thoughts and feelings in order that they might be better able to assist their relative in need. The person of the pastor is often symbolic in these crisis consultations. He or she represents safety and support; persons in need look to the Church for assurance and guidance in times of great stress.

For some parents, the communication about AIDS and homosexuality is experienced as threatening. It may confront deeply held beliefs and normative principles of morality of the parent, spouse, or sibling. Because these beliefs and morals are judged to be of the essence of a person's life, they can serve as a block to communication and relationship with a relative whose lifestyle may have departed from these expressed norms. It is not easy for family members to process alone these conflicting thoughts and feelings. Pastors are often thought of as allies, as persons who share compatible values with family members. They are considered the moral teachers, representing the ethical and religious values that have given meaning to the principles that guide people's lives. It is understandable why parents and others in crisis seek the counsel of pastors.

It was within this context that Brenda and Harry Searles sought the counsel of Rabbi Miklowitz. They were members of Congregation Beth El and were active participants in the temple's programs. The Searles were owners of a large and successful restaurant which their oldest son, Jeffrey, managed. Two days prior to their meeting with the rabbi, they had returned from a visit with their youngest son, Len, who had been hospitalized in San Francisco with Pneumocystis pneumonia.

The Searles were visibly upset when they entered Rabbi Miklowitz's office. Harry spoke for the couple. He told the rabbi that he and Brenda had not slept very much for the past two weeks since they first learned that their son was seriously ill in California. They had flown to San Francisco to be with him, and were shocked to discover that he was gay and that he had AIDS. Harry's voice began to break as he pronounced those two words, "gay" and "AIDS." Brenda was not successful in fighting back her tears.

As the rabbi listened, Harry continued: "We have not been able to tell the other children about Len. They know he is ill, but they don't know what's wrong. We told them he had a serious respiratory problem, but nothing more." At this point Brenda interjected: "Rabbi, it will tear the family apart." Harry nodded affirmatively: "The doctors told us that he would need assistance. Naturally, we would like him to come home. But our small community is not ready for this. People wouldn't understand. I told Brenda that it would probably ruin our business."

Brenda looked away as her husband finished his last statement. The rabbi asked her if there was something she wanted to say. Brenda began to sob deeply, and through her tears she said, "Rabbi, he's our son, and I fear that he is dying. We can't abandon him, even if it means a loss of business. Every time Harry and I talk about this, we get stuck on this point. I'm very angry at him for placing his reputation and business success above Len's need for his family at this time. That's the reason we have come to talk with you."

Harry was silent. He told the rabbi how difficult it was to make this first move to consult with him. The couple admitted their embarrassment in telling the rabbi that their son was gay and that he was seriously ill with AIDS. Rabbi Miklowitz was empathetic and caring. He reached out his arms and held Brenda's and Harry's hands. They were visibly moved by the expression of support and the words the rabbi spoke to them in response.

Rabbi Miklowitz counseled the Searles that they needed to communicate openly with the rest of the immediate family. He told them that Len needed the understanding, love, and support of his entire family. The parents, he advised, were needlessly carrying the whole burden alone. The couple confessed that they did not feel able to tell their children, and asked if the rabbi could help them in this difficult task.

Recognizing the difficulties both Brenda and Harry were experiencing as they anticipated this communication with their other children and their spouses, the rabbi agreed to facilitate the encounter in the temple's meeting room. The Searles, though apprehensive, seemed relieved that the rabbi would mediate this difficult communication with the rest of the family. Before they left his office, the rabbi helped the couple to clarify their desires with respect to Len's future care. It was clear that despite the anticipated problems, they both wanted to invite their son to return home. Brenda was most adamant on this point; Harry, although tentative, was in agreement.

The meeting took place on the following Thursday evening. With the exception of Jeffrey's wife, all of the Searles' children and their spouses were present. Jeffrey, thirty-four, was the oldest. He and Sandra were married and had two children, Jonathan and Terri. Charles, thirty-one, was married to Anne and had one child, Sarah. Barbara, twenty-eight, engaged to Peter Gluck and intending to be married the following autumn, was an accountant. Len, twenty-six, the youngest of the Searles' children, had graduated with a master's degree in business administration and had completed an advanced program in hotel management. At the time of his diagnosis he had been working for a large hotel chain, and was the assistant general manager of one of the company's properties in San Francisco.

Rabbi Miklowitz began the meeting by thanking the family members for gathering. He clarified his role in facilitating this meeting, acknowledging that their parents needed to talk with them about some important family concerns, and wished to do so with his support. He told the family that he and their parents had met previously and that the present gathering was the result of that prior conversation.

Harry Searles then spoke: "Your brother, Len, is more seriously ill than your mother and I were able to admit to you. He has AIDS. His doctors have advised us that he will need some assistance. Mother and I wish to bring him home and care for him here." Brenda nodded affirmatively, but remained silent.

Jeffrey was the first to speak. He was clearly agitated by the news and asked a series of rapid-fire questions. "AIDS? Does that mean Len's gay? That's a 'gay disease,' isn't it? Is he dying? How come we didn't know sooner?" The room was silent.

Rabbi Miklowitz looked at Harry and Brenda who signaled that he should attempt to respond to some of the issues raised by Jeffrey's questions. The rabbi affirmed that their younger brother was gay, and had recently shared this personal information with his parents. The rabbi continued by explaining that while AIDS affected a significantly larger percentage of gay men, it was not a gay disease, nor was it easy to contract the disease through ordinary contact with an infected person. Len had been ill for some months before his hospitalization. His current medical status was guarded; he was not fully responsive to the treatments for pneumonia, although his doctors were hopeful that they would be able to manage his infection. Although not in imminent danger of dying, Len would need support which the family could best provide.

Jeffrey was uncomfortable as the rabbi was speaking. It was clear that he was not convinced that Len's return was in the best general interest of the family. However, he was reluctant to verbalize his opinions. Charles and Anne sat together; she was holding her husband's hand while he spoke: "I think we should certainly offer to help Len, and if he wants to come back home, then, as far as we're concerned, he's welcome." Barbara spoke next, affirming what Charles said. She told the family that she had known for some time about Len's homosexuality. Len had shared this information with her. She did not tell others in the family what her brother told her, feeling that the family was not ready to deal with the information. Barbara was the closest member of the family to Len, and seemed more upset that her younger brother had not communicated about his medical problems directly with her.

The rabbi helped the family to talk about these and many other issues that evening, and together to plan how they would express their support and love for their son and brother. The rabbi pledged his continuing support for the Searles family. Harry and Brenda were visibly relieved that the whole family had participated in the meeting with Rabbi Miklowitz. The family was understanding and supportive of their decision to invite their son to return home so that he could benefit from their care. Len was greatly comforted by the telephone call from his parents, and was particularly moved when his father told him, "Len, we all love you, and we do not want you to be alone. Please come home and let us help you battle this thing together." Len said, "Dad, I love you all, and I want to be with you."

During the next several months before Len's death, Rabbi

Miklowitz was very helpful to various members of the Searles family. He was continually supportive of the family, and helped other members of the congregation to reach out to them. Len's return to his family and community was a time of growth not only for the Searles, but for many other people in the community who were strengthened by the example of a family's loving concern for their sick son and brother. Len died surrounded by the acceptance and love of a family who survived the dual crisis of confronting simultaneously a family member's homosexuality and life-threatening illness.

Herbert Moore's family was similarly supportive. Stephanie decided to tell her oldest son and his family during a planned visit with them in Phoenix. She wanted to tell Rob in person, and this trip coincided with Herbert's revelation to her. With the help of a priest in whom she confided, Stephanie prepared for the discussion. She told her son the story in a private conversation. Later he shared the news with his wife, and together they expressed their understanding and support for their parents. Rob called his father and verbalized this support. Herbert was comforted by his son's words.

It was Stephanie who also told the couple's two daughters. They were more visibly upset by the communication, although one of them acknowledged that she had long suspected that her father might have been involved in homosexual activities. Stephanie delayed telling the youngest daughter, afraid that she would fall apart with the news. Stephanie's priest advisor counseled her not to delay the communication. He reasoned that the youngest daughter might resent the delay, be angry that she was not informed immediately, and become distrustful that something else might be withheld from her. Stephanie agreed.

The communication with the last of the Moore children actually was accelerated because Herbert developed a high fever and pneumonia which necessitated his hospitalization. Both of his daughters responded lovingly to their father, assuring him of their acceptance and support. Herbert told his youngest, "I don't deserve your love." She countered, "Of course you do, Daddy, of course you do. We *all* love you, and always will."

Bearing the Burdens of Caring for
a Person with AIDS

Like other chronic, life-threatening illnesses, AIDS makes enormous demands upon the physical and emotional reserves of persons with the disease and those who assist in their care. Family members who assume the role and functions of principal care-providers soon realize the effects the disease has on them. Some persons with AIDS, especially those individuals unable to provide for many of their own basic needs, become utterly dependent upon others. It is not uncommon that the major responsibility for providing basic assistance is borne by one or two family members or friends.

The two cases we shall review underscore some of the problems that care-providers experience in assisting an individual with AIDS. In the first case, we shall consider the problems of a spouse who assists her hemophiliac husband during his two-year battle with the disease, and in the second case we shall focus on the experiences of a gay man who cares for a dying lover. In both cases, we shall consider pastoral care opportunities in which the Church can reach out to support the helpers.

Norm was thirty-one when he was diagnosed with AIDS in 1982, causing a tremendous shock to his family. His bizarre symptoms of a malfunctioning immune system had baffled the physicians who attempted to diagnose his condition. The number of helper T-cells was decreased as well as the ratio of T-4 to T-8 cells. He had abnormal skin test responses, increased immunoglobulins, and defective natural killer cell activity. As a result, Norm was vulnerable to a variety of serious infections and other diseases. At the time of his diagnosis, there was a paucity of knowledge about AIDS, and even less understanding of its epidemiology among hemophiliacs who were regularly treated with Factor VIII concentrate, a blood-clotting protein derived from donor blood plasma. Norm was a lifelong hemophiliac and had received Factor VIII treatments to prevent the recurrence of bleeding.

Norm and Claudia had been married in 1977. The couple had grown up in different parts of the country. Norm was a native of New Hampshire, while Claudia was raised in Chicago.

They had met at the Wharton School where both were pursuing advanced graduate degrees in business. They were a typical young professional couple engaged in dual careers. In their long-range plan, they intended to postpone childbearing activity for several years while they concentrated on the development of their respective careers. Norm commuted to New York City each day from Stamford, Connecticut. Claudia had a job in Stamford where the couple had purchased a luxury condominium. Until Norm became ill in 1982, their lives were uncomplicated and were proceeding according to their plans.

Claudia experienced many difficulties as she attempted to cope with Norm's multiple AIDS-related illnesses. Apart from family and a few close friends in whom she could confide, Claudia felt emotionally isolated. Before his diagnosis was confirmed, Norm had been ill, requiring many brief periods of sick leave. These unexplained illnesses were distressing, requiring Claudia to take time away from her job to take care of Norm.

When he was diagnosed, Norm became depressed and angry. He was emotionally volatile, frequently addressing his verbal assaults at Claudia. She was understanding, but nonetheless felt victimized by his unpredictable moodiness. Their apartment, though spacious, seemed small and restrictive. As Norm's health progressively deteriorated, they were forced to spend more time together in this setting.

Reluctantly, Norm agreed to permit the local hospice program to assist Claudia in his care. In the earliest days of his illness he would allow no one except Claudia to assist him. The hospice program became very important for Claudia as well as for Norm. It provided her with some individuals who both understood her concerns and were willing to respond to them.

Through the hospice program, the Conants met Father Arthur Lyons. Father Lyons was a member of the hospice team, providing pastoral assistance to families caring for a terminally ill member. Norm and Claudia were both Roman Catholics, although not active members of a parish community at the time when Norm became ill. Father Lyons visited the Conants in their apartment and over the course of several months developed a good relationship with both Norm and Claudia.

Adjustments in Sexual Relationship

There were many issues that Norm and Claudia discussed with Father Lyons, individually and together as a couple. Claudia was hesitant at first to talk about her changing sexual relationship with Norm. After Norm's diagnosis, Claudia had been tested for the presence of AIDS antibodies and was found to be seronegative. Since their marriage, she had used a diaphragm in conjunction with a spermicidal foam as a method of contraception. In retrospect, she credits this protective barrier as the way she avoided becoming infected with a virus that neither she nor Norm was aware he was carrying.

As a result of Norm's illness, the couple had to make changes in their sexual practices which both found to be difficult. Father Lyons was very understanding and helpful as Claudia and Norm worked through some of the difficulties in adjusting their sexual life.

Norm seemed less interested in sex than Claudia, although Claudia expressed initial apprehensions about feeling vulnerable to infection. When Norm and Claudia spoke together with Father Lyons, Norm said that he refrained from sexual relations for many reasons. Sometimes he simply did not feel well. At other times the medications he was taking seemed to weaken his sexual desires. The most serious obstacles, in Norm's opinion, were the feelings of guilt or frustration about seeking sexual pleasures with Claudia, fearing potential risks to her health. At the same time, he admitted that he often felt the need for her physical support, and the sense of security that physical intimacy with her provided.

Father Lyons encouraged Norm and Claudia to experiment with new ways of enjoying sex that would be compatible with her safety and Norm's physical needs and limitations. Claudia admitted that her needs for physical intimacy were great and that she very much wanted to have a child with Norm (although she admitted that this was too risky), and she realized that Norm shared these same needs. Father Lyons was responsive to their expressed concerns, and encouraged Norm and Claudia to work to find mutually satisfying and pleasurable ways of engaging in sexual activities. He helped the couple to be honest with each other about their frustrations and disappointments with their attempts to modify their sexual behaviors.

Claudia remarked that Norm seemed less depressed as they began to communicate more openly about their sexual relationship, and they both grew more relaxed as they explored ways of enjoying intimate pleasures together. Father Lyons had counseled them to maintain a sense of humor as they attempted to make the necessary adjustments in their sexual behaviors. Both Claudia and Norm often laughed that it was a priest who was the person most helpful to them in working out the tensions in this important aspect of their relationship. They often referred to Lyons as *their* "Dr. Ruth," a celebrity sex therapist.

Patient Care "Burnout"

Claudia was devoted to Norm's care. From the time of his diagnosis until his death in 1984, Norm was hospitalized on four separate occasions. Apart from these hospitalizations, Norm remained at home with Claudia. In the final seven months of his illness, Norm was unable to work and became even more dependent upon Claudia for assistance. It was during this phase of his illness that he accepted the support of the hospice care team.

As noted above, this was a reluctant decision on Norm's part. He wanted Claudia with him, and wanted her to provide directly the care he required. When she was away from him, during the work day or during periods when she sought a respite from providing care, Norm was despondent. Hospice volunteers noted his agitation and hesitancy to allow them to do some ordinary things for him. Often he would say, "When Claudia comes back, she will take care of that."

Until Claudia began to receive help from the hospice program, she did not have anyone with whom she felt she could talk about the emotional burdens she was experiencing in caring for Norm. Her mother who lived in Chicago was somewhat helpful to her, and they talked regularly on the telephone. But her mother betrayed an Italo-American cultural bias which sees the role of the wife in a totally self-giving position to her husband. Claudia's sense of obligation to Norm not only was reinforced by her mother, but also was intensified by the fact that Norm had contracted AIDS through his necessary dependence upon blood products to prevent bleeding. In her mind he was an innocent victim; the least she could do as his wife was to provide total care for him.

The kind of care she wanted to provide for Norm and the actual additional energies she expended in doing these things were taking their toll on Claudia. In addition to working at a demanding job, she was rushing home each day at noon to prepare lunch and spend the time with Norm. This was possible because her office was only ten minutes' commuting time from their condominium. Norm looked forward to her return, and was agitated on those days when her schedule did not permit this midday visit. He was very upset when she had to be away over-night for a business trip, and Claudia tried to curtail her business travel as much as possible. Her employers, sensitive to her family concerns, were flexible in arranging her travel schedule, and were supportive when she required some extra time in order to take care of Norm in the morning or during the day.

She called him at least two or three times during the work day to reassure him and to check up on him. His needs were always on her mind. As Norm's dependency increased and his body grew weaker, Claudia gradually began to realize that he was going to die from this disease. In the beginning, they adopted the attitude that we are going to beat this thing. Norm actually said that he thought he would be the first hemophiliac to beat AIDS.

Now that hope was dim, although Claudia did not want to admit that to Norm. She was beginning to accept the reality of his decline. Acceptance of this fact was not easy, and it came into her consciousness at times when she felt herself most vul-nerable. One afternoon while she was at the office, the thought that Norm would die flooded her awareness and she began to cry. It frightened her to admit that her feelings were not under her direct control. She tried to hold back her tears, but was unable to do so. Alone in her office, she sobbed and wept.

In her next conversation with Father Lyons, Claudia began to talk about the burdens she was carrying. Father Lyons under-stood what was happening to Norm and to Claudia. He said to her, "Claudia, you have to start paying more attention to yourself." She recalls the old cliché he used: "God helps those who help themselves." As Claudia and the priest talked, she reminisced about the day she and Norm were married and the words of the vows they pronounced: "For better or worse, in sickness and in health, to love and to cherish, until death do us part." Claudia admitted that she never thought that she would have to honor the darker side of that commitment so early in their relationship. Father Lyons was clearly touched by the depth of her commitment to Norm, but cautioned that her sense of duty to be with him and care for him could burn her out. She needed to take care of herself as well as Norm.

Through Father Lyons' help and with the support of a nurse in the hospice care program assisting the Conants, Claudia became active in a group sponsored by the AIDS Action Committee for the families of persons with AIDS. Through that group Claudia found the insight and support she needed. The group also was helpful in providing valuable suggestions about practical care-related concerns. Although the group began to take over some of the functions that her individual conversations with Father Lyons had previously supplied, she nonetheless continued to talk with him. Their meetings became less concerned with emotional issues, and more focused on spiritual needs. Father Lyons was able to help Claudia to express her concerns in shared prayer. Claudia began to pray together with Norm, and they found that this activity was comforting and brought them closer together.

Fran and Michael had been lovers for four years when Fran became ill and was diagnosed with AIDS. With the increasing incidence of AIDS among gay men, in 1984 both Fran and Michael had decided to be tested, and both were reported as seropositive. For more than a year after testing neither of the men showed any symptoms. In December of 1985, Fran developed Pneumocystis carinii pneumonia. Qualifying for an experimental drug protocol being administered in a New York hospital, Fran was hopeful that his life expectancy might be extended and the quality of his life improved. During 1986, and until his death in February 1987, Michael was his most dependable support and companion.

Fran and Michael were both Roman Catholics. Fran had not

been a practicing Catholic until he met Michael. Michael was an active participant in a Dignity chapter, a support group for gay and lesbian Catholics. Fran and Michael attended a weekly celebration of the Eucharist on Sunday evenings in a New York church. Through this involvement they became friendly with Father Bob Clarke, a Jesuit priest who ministered to homosexual persons. When Fran became ill, Michael, himself a former seminarian, immediately called Father Bob for support. During the next fourteen months, Michael and Fran often sought the help of Father Bob for a variety of needs.

From the outset of Fran's diagnosis, Michael was determined that he would remain with his lover and care for him. Both Fran and Michael knew of friends who had separated when one of the partners became ill. Michael was resolved that he would not abandon Fran, and Fran was relieved and grateful for the strength of Michael's love and determination. However, Michael did not realize how much this commitment would require of him in terms of physical and emotional energy. Without the assistance he received from other friends, family, and medical support personnel, he would not have been able to meet Fran's increasing needs for care.

Michael's job as a commercial artist gave him enough flexibility in scheduling that he was able to be at home with Fran whenever Fran's health required greater support. Michael had a studio area in their loft apartment which permitted him to do some of his work at home. As Fran's illness progressed, Michael found himself having to spend more and more time at home.

Financial Worries

Father Clarke was an important sounding-board for Michael. Knowing how sensitive Fran was to many things about his disease, Michael tried not to burden him additionally with his own frustrations. Michael called Father Bob his "safety valve," a way of releasing some of the pressures building up within him. Among the concerns Michael expressed were worries about finances. Both he and Fran had excellent jobs, and had been able to obtain a mortgage on their loft apartment in

Greenwich Village. When Fran became unable to work regularly, there were major disruptions in their income, since a significant portion of Fran's salary was linked to sales commissions. Michael began to assume an unequal portion of their expenses, and this was a source of increasing concern for him.

Fran, too, was worried about financial management, how they would be able to meet their ordinary expenses, and how they would be able to pay for increasing costs associated with Fran's physical care. Fran would often raise the issue with Michael who tended to dismiss his friend's worries as not important. What Michael failed to recognize was that Fran's self-esteem was negatively affected by his inability to work and to contribute. Father Bob was instrumental in pointing this out to Michael and it helped him better to appreciate some of Fran's outbursts and frustrations.

Michael encouraged Fran to find out about disability benefits for which he might be eligible. As his health worsened and he was not able to work at all, he was eligible for permanent disability status, and qualified for supplemental income that brought his total benefit payments to about seventy-five percent of his former salary base. This eased some of the tensions. The fact that he qualified and was participating in an experimental treatment program took away a great deal of the financial concerns about medical costs associated with AIDS.

Spiritual Growth

Michael found a considerable amount of support from his participation in a faith community. Throughout the ordeal of living with Fran during his battle with AIDS, Michael continued to worship each Sunday. While he was able, Fran continued to participate as well. As friends within the community died of AIDS, they found themselves attending an increasing number of funerals and memorial services. Fran said that he found a lot of hope and comfort in his faith, and Michael agreed.

Father Bob encouraged Michael to bring the Eucharist home to his friend when Fran was unable to attend Mass. Michael was deeply moved by this suggestion and quickly responded to the priest's initiative. After Fran's death, Michael confessed that these times of sharing the Eucharist with his sick friend were among the most important memories he cherished.

On two occasions, Father Bob celebrated the Eucharist in Fran and Michael's apartment. One of these times, he administered the sacrament of the sick. Michael's sister and her husband and Fran's mother and brother were also present for this occasion. The family members brought casseroles and Michael prepared a special dessert. All of them enjoyed a potluck supper after the liturgy, and Fran, though somewhat weakened, was visibly comforted by the religious and social aspects of the evening. He felt well enough to play a couple of pieces on his guitar, and everyone appreciated his added effort. It was his own special contribution.

One evening when Father Bob stopped by to visit, Fran raised the issue of his own death and wanted to talk together with Michael and the priest about his requests for his funeral. Michael was surprised to hear Fran raise this concern, since he had never discussed the topic previously. Father Bob was immediately responsive to the suggestion and was helpful as he encouraged Fran to proceed with the agenda.

Fran was very much at peace as he acknowledged the fact that he was dying. He said he wished that he could live longer, but that he was ready to face his own death. He was able to thank Michael for being so faithful to him, and for helping him in every way. Several nights before he died, in Father Bob's presence, Fran told Michael that without his example and support, he would never have rediscovered his relationship with God. He admitted that his faith made facing AIDS and his death bearable. He wanted his funeral liturgy to reflect his belief in the triumph of life over death.

He had selected some passages in the paperback edition of the Bible that Father Bob had given him some months before. He had folded down the corners of the pages of those texts he wished to be read during his funeral. Michael was moved as Fran spoke about his death, his faith, his consolation. Father Bob allowed Fran to speak uninterruptedly. When Fran was finished, Father Bob took the Bible from his hands, and began to read aloud the passages that Fran had indicated. When he concluded the readings, he paused and invited Fran and Michael to join with him in prayer. The priest began to pray, using the themes suggested by the scriptural texts. Fran and Michael voiced their own prayers. Not only was this experience helpful to Fran who sensed a need to talk about his death and funeral, but it was comforting to Michael as well.

Michael found these various spiritual experiences to be meaningful. However, he continued to search for spiritual significance in Fran's physical struggles and in the lives of so many others with AIDS whom he knew. In his monograph, *AIDS: The Spiritual Dilemma* (1987), John Fortunato makes an attempt to express the meaning he sees in the lives of persons with AIDS.

> So lacking a reasonable answer, I will make a stab at a *nonrational* answer to the why of AIDS. And it is this. If our journey with AIDS serves to bring us all home to the grand and grave, the joyful and sobering truth of our mortality; if this suffering helps heal the madness of an eternally empty later whose existence we have duped ourselves into believing in; if this nightmare brings back to our consciousness the resurrection hope without which life is just so much courageous despair, then in this groaning of creation, with tears and sighs, perhaps the Holy Spirit will usher in some modicum of peace or even a corner of salvation that might otherwise have been unattainable. And in that travail, perhaps . . . perhaps we will glimpse the meaning of AIDS for our spiritual journey. (pp. 85–86)

As Michael searched for his own personal meaning, stretching his faith in ways he had not experienced before Fran's illness, Father Bob was an important resource. Michael benefited from their conversations which frequently involved issues of faith and meaning. Clarke did not attempt to provide answers to unanswerable questions. He encouraged Michael to seek his own answers in his prayer and reflection. Michael found much consolation in scriptural meditation which Clarke fostered and encouraged.

On one occasion, when Michael was preoccupied with the amount of suffering that Fran was experiencing, Father Clarke suggested that he reflect upon the text in 1 Corinthians 12. In that chapter St. Paul speaks about the varieties of gifts and ministries within the Christian community. Despite their diversity, the same God is present and at work in all of them. The spiritual gifts are meant to be God's response to the needs of his people. At times, God empowers a person to be a healer (1 Cor 12:9); at other times, the Lord gives a person the ability to help another to bear sufferings and grow through these experiences. In his care for his sick friend, Michael was helping Fran to bear his sufferings and to find meaning in them. In this situation, Michael was an instrument of God's healing. God's healing touch was being mediated through Michael's fidelity, companionship, love, and care. Far from being distant or absent, God was present in a healing way in the midst of human suffering.

Clarke was always supportive and affirming. The priest did not avoid the difficult questions, nor gloss over Fran's or Michael's real concerns. He did not propose facile solutions to complex problems. He relied on the resources of Scripture and prayer in ministering to both men. He searched for meaning alongside them, and by his presence signaled that he was willing to share the journey. This seemed to be everything that Fran and Michael were asking in their relationship with him.

Concerns for One's Own Survival

Although Michael had remained healthy despite his own verified exposure to the virus, he was preparing himself for the possibility that he too might become ill. The fact that Fran was dying precipitated a host of concerns in Michael. He began to speak more often about the possibility that he, too, would become ill. Living through Fran's illness made him aware of the pain and suffering a person with AIDS endures. He wondered who would care for him should he become ill. He had been there for Fran, but feared that no one would be there for him. He knew that his family would support him, but he was unhappy with the prospect of the burden that such care would place upon them.

Father Bob anticipated Michael's concerns and occasionally would ask some direct questions. "Are you worried about getting sick yourself?" These simple inquiries helped Michael to voice his fears and concerns, and simply talking about them seemed to help in their management. Michael expressed guilt that Fran was dying while he, at present, was symptom-free. Neither blamed the other for having the virus, and there was never direct discussion between them about who infected whom. However, Michael felt sure that it was only a matter of time before he developed ARC or AIDS. The thought of becoming sick while Fran was still alive or after he died was chilling.

Father Bob suggested that Michael participate in a support group sponsored by the Gay Men's Health Crisis in New York City. The group was organized to respond to the special needs of family members and friends who were providing direct care for persons with AIDS. Michael accepted this suggestion and found the group helpful with some issues. Other things he decided he would have to resolve on his own. In all of these self-explorations, Michael sensed the support of his friend, Father Bob Clarke. He said that the priest was "a light in the shadows," like the "reassuring presence of a parent to a child who is frightened by the darkness of night."

A Pastor's Reflection

BettyClare Moffatt cites the case of Steve Peters, a gay minister with AIDS, in her book *When Someone You Love Has AIDS* (1986). Peters was diagnosed with Kaposi's sarcoma and lymphoma in 1982. He reflected upon his illness and the spiritual meanings he was drawing from those experiences. The following is excerpted from his recorded interview with Moffatt.

> *What does this tell me? It is my personal belief that God is giving me enough time to do what needs to be done in my life. I have a strong faith in God and His plan for my life. . . .*

> *I feel at peace about where I am now and where I am going and what I have to say. You see, before I got AIDS, I was trying to minister, trying to help others, but I really couldn't. I started waking up when AIDS hit. To me AIDS is an incredible gift of awakening. It has helped me to realize my own sense of self and what I have to give. . . . I am still a Christian; I am a man, a minister, who has AIDS, that's all. . . .*

Before I got AIDS, I often felt that nobody loved me. Now there's not as much need for one person; I can reach out to so many friends. . . . I feel that God has told me that I can't keep love until I give it away. In fact, what I feel is that I, Steve Peters, am now scared into life *instead of being scared to death. And I thank God for this every day. (pp. 72–74)*

The privilege of ministering to persons with AIDS and to their family and friends awakens one to life. Serious and terminal illness has a way of catalyzing the kinds of experiences that Steve Peters describes. It has that effect on the dying person. It has the same potential power for awakening those who assist in the care of someone who is facing death. Pastors are formed by their experiences and grow as a result of them. AIDS makes demands on patients, family, and friends and on those who reach out to assist them as pastors. Such encounters may be occasions for personal and spiritual growth for the pastor as well as for those he or she attempts to serve. In each of these encounters we are reminded of the words of St. Paul in his Letter to the Romans: "Now we know that for those who love God all things work together unto good" (Rom 8:28). God's healing touches the healer as well as the afflicted. One is ministered to by the very persons to whom one extends a helping hand.

8

Grief and Bereavement

Grief is an integral component of all human relationships. Whenever we love and care for another person, we invest parts of ourselves in that person. This may involve the commitment of physical and material resources, the sharing of possessions, time, and experiences. Relationships also involve emotional, psychological, and spiritual investments. The intensity, strength, and duration of these bonds affect the experiences of loss when the relationship is interrupted or broken.

Death is an ultimate experience of loss. It severs many aspects of human attachments and precipitates grieving. The survivor is faced with the work of withdrawing energies invested in activities and relationships formerly shared with the deceased. The language of bonding is universally employed to describe the various levels of attachment that exist in all human relationships. If *bonding* describes the process of building relationships, then *unbonding* represents the work of grieving.

Freud used the term *decathexis* when speaking about human grieving. By this term he meant the disengagement and gradual withdrawal of the psychic energies formerly invested in the lost relationship. He assumed that a person had to complete the work of grieving before he or she would be free to make new investments in other relationships. In this understanding of grieving, the survivor is faced with specific tasks that require work and time to complete. The primary agenda involves release from the aspects of the relationship that involved bonding. The second task involves adjustment to living without the lost relationship. The resolution of the process entails the formation of new relationships and the psychological investment in these relationships.

Grieving is an important and necessary part of facing experiences of loss, and real work is essential if a survivor is to be able to make healthy reinvestments in other relationships. The process of normal grieving is genuine work. Some people fail to consider this seriously when dealing with situations of loss. When we speak of work, we generally understand that energies are committed to a certain project or activity in order to accomplish some specified goal. In this context grieving is appropriately described as work. A griever requires social and emotional supports to accomplish this work in order to be able later to invest his or her physical and emotional resources in other works. Too often we expect that grief takes care of itself. We appeal to the aphorism that "time heals all." Time is an indispensable component of grieving. However, time alone does not heal. A bereaved person must assume an active role in the work of grieving. He or she must become engaged in a number of activities that help in resolving the loss.

In this final chapter we shall consider some experiences of grief and bereavement associated with AIDS, and how survivors are actively involving themselves in the resolution of their losses. Among care-providers, pastors are in especially privileged positions to facilitate, encourage, and assist persons facing loss and those who survive them. Pastoral care plays important functional roles in the work of grieving. However, for pastoral interventions to be maximally effective, pastors need to be attentive to the physical and psychological dimensions of the work of grieving, as well as to the spiritual. In all of our examples we shall focus on practical cases where pastors can be helpful in supporting the essential work of grieving.

What Does the Relationship Mean?

In our common parlance, we routinely describe relationships as unique. By this we imply that there is a rare and unusual combination of experiences that describe one person's relationship with another. Although other persons may share aspects of those experiences in common, each relationship is distinct. This is evident in family life. Each child enjoys a unique relationship with parents and siblings. Affectional bonds, expressions of intimacy, levels of sharing, and forms of dependencies differ, subtly or dramatically, in each of these relationships. To understand what the loss means to a grieving individual, one must appreciate the aspects of the bond which made it unique.

It is important to bring the same understanding to bear when one encounters situations of loss associated with AIDS. The following case of a nineteen year old HIV-positive, intravenous drug user hospitalized with a serious hepatitis B infection illustrates this point.

Greg is the only child of Sheila and Don Logan. The Logans are a middle-class working family who live in a comfortable suburban home. Greg was educated in a private secondary school. After graduation he began college in a large public university, but dropped out after his first year. Sheila and Don suspected that Greg was involved in drugs, but they were unwilling to admit how deeply his habits were affecting not only his academic and social behaviors, but also his health.

When Greg was hospitalized with a fulminating Hepatitis B infection, he was severely jaundiced. He responded poorly to aggressive curative treatments. Early in the course of diagnosis and treatment, it was discovered that he was HIV-positive and his body immune response was weak. The physicians attending him felt that his chance of surviving the liver infection were minimal. They felt that it was important to alert Greg's parents to the distinct possibility that he would die.

Sheila was very attached to her son. In some ways she shared more of herself with Greg than she did with her husband, Don. From the time Greg was a baby, she spent considerable time with him, talking and sharing experiences with him. Throughout his school years, Sheila was always home, engaging Greg in conversations about his interests and activities. She found it difficult when Greg began to pull away from her during high school. They had some heated arguments as he attempted to exercise his independence. Sheila found it particularly difficult when Greg left for college. When he decided to drop out at the end of his freshman year he moved into an apartment with some of his friends. He visited his parents' home infrequently.

Don, on the other hand, seemed distant from his son. By disposition, Don was a quiet man. He worked as a plumber, maintaining his own business from his home. Sheila was his business manager and bookkeeper, affording her the opportunity to remain at home while being employed. Don seemed to tacitly accept the relationship Sheila fostered with Greg, and felt absolved from direct involvement with many of the decisions of child-rearing. As a result, Greg and Don did not have a close, personal father-son relationship.

When Greg was hospitalized, both Sheila and Don turned to their minister for support. Moderately active participants in their Congregational parish, the Logans called Rev. Buckingham when the doctors told them of Greg's prognosis. They were alarmed by the news that Greg might have contracted AIDS through his drug involvements. Knowing this, they were frightened by the doctor's guarded statements that Greg might not survive his serious liver infection. And should he survive, would he go on to develop AIDS and die soon after? These were the concerns the Logans brought to Rev. Buckingham.

Although Sheila and Don attended services regularly, their pastor did not know the family well. He came to know them at the time of their crisis. He had never met Greg until he visited him in the hospital. During that visit he soon realized that Greg's doctors had discussed openly their judgments about his worsening health. Greg was alert, although weak. Greg told the minister in a matter-of-fact manner that he "might not make it." "I've got a pretty bad case of hepatitis, and the doctors also think I might have AIDS."

Buckingham had learned these basic facts from the Logans before he met with Greg, but was relieved that the doctors had communicated openly about these issues with Greg. Rev. Buckingham spent the first visit with Greg helping him to explore his feelings about the information that he was gradually absorbing. Greg seemed able to talk about the facts of his diagnosis, but, apart from the single comment about "not making it," Greg did not make any other reference to dying.

Rev. Buckingham met with the parents several times. In a

private meeting with Sheila, he was able to assess her needs more clearly than during his initial meeting with the couple. Sheila was frightened by what the doctors had told her, even though she was unwilling to believe that Greg would die. She felt confident that he would rally and recover. However, there were other indications that helped Buckingham to realize that she had heard the message the physicians were trying to communicate.

Sheila was not sleeping well, and since Greg's hospitalization she had lost several pounds. She and her husband were having serious difficulties talking. Sheila confessed that "Don and I don't have the kind of relationship where we can talk things out." She was feeling alone in this crisis. Buckingham was the first person with whom she was able to ventilate some of her feelings. Much of the language she used during their conversation revolved around words like "loss" and "lonely." "At nights, I lay awake in bed, feeling cold and lonely, like a person who has lost everything," Sheila said. She emphasized that Don was a good man, but incapable of dealing with problems. "He doesn't know what to do for Greg, and he doesn't know what to do for me."

When Buckingham met alone with Don, he got a different picture. Don was quite able to express his feelings. He felt guilty that he had not been more involved in Greg's life as his son was growing up. Now he felt impotent to interact in any significant way with Greg. Don said he felt that his wife was not doing well with the knowledge about Greg's condition and that she was unwilling to accept the fact that Greg would probably die. "He's been her whole life, Reverend. I don't know what she's going to do when he is gone." Don acknowledged that he and his wife did not have a "good talking relationship." He admitted that he tended to be quiet and private. He hastened to add that he had told Rev. Buckingham more in their meeting than he had been able to share with his wife in years.

What Rev. Buckingham learned from these pastoral visits and conversations with the Logans were some of the issues that would contribute to the ways in which they would face loss. Sheila and Don attached different meanings to Greg's diagnosis and his probable death. To minister effectively to this family in this crisis required knowledge and the ability to respond to the different ways in which the anticipated loss was experienced.

Anticipatory Grieving

For many people a diagnosis of AIDS represents a physical and psychological challenge to survive as well as a spiritual and emotional preparation for death. It is on these latter issues that we shall focus our attention. In their attempts to understand the ways in which people cope with the knowledge that they will die, mental health professionals have described a process called *anticipatory grieving*. As the term suggests, anticipatory grieving is a behavioral pattern related to an awareness of an impending loss, to its physical and psychological impact, and to the ways in which emotional attachments to the dying person are gradually released. Anticipatory grieving is presumed to attenuate the negative effects of loss. It functions as a psychological buffer both for the dying person and for those who will survive the death of a loved one.

Knowledge that death is approaching sets in motion disengagement dynamics. Difficult as it is to begin to separate from the physical and psychological attachments we have formed with a loved person, the fact of approaching death necessitates preparation for an ultimate separation. As we stated at the beginning of this chapter, when a loved one dies, survivors attempt to adjust to the multiple losses associated with the death. This is the normal and necessary work of grieving.

This work, however, may begin prior to the actual death of a loved one. To a degree, the processes of grieving can be anticipated. In the case of a dying person who is aware of his or her impending death, this is an ordinary part of preparation for death. For survivors, anticipatory grieving can help them to prepare for the loss and cushion some painful aspects of the loss.

Anticipatory grieving is not without its inherent liabilities. In cases of AIDS where the terminal period may be of considerable duration, lasting for many months, it is possible that some persons could complete the grief work prior to the loved one's actual death. The implications for this are immediately obvious. Grieving has a predictable and time-limited course. Dying persons frequently express fears that they will die alone and abandoned. If those who are closest to them complete their grieving prior to a loved one's actual death, there is the possibility that the dying person will sense the emotional distancing and disengagement. This may be perceived as rejection and abandonment.

It is reasonable to assume that persons with AIDS and those individuals who are closest to them will utilize the period between definitive diagnosis and death to prepare for the separation. In addition to involvement with practical concerns of reviewing one's estate, preparing or updating one's will, and indicating one's desires about funeral and burial arrangements, a dying person is also concerned about reaching closure on aspects of interpersonal relationships.

An important part of preparing to die is saying goodbye to people who have been important in one's life. Some of these farewells can be accomplished easily; others require greater time and effort. This is true both for the dying person and for those individuals who share some relationship with him or her. The amount of grief and its intensity are proportionate to the value one person may have for the other. For example, a lover of eight months may have stronger emotional bonds to a dying gay man than his blood brother may feel. The knowledge, openness, and communication between a dying person and important individuals within his or her social network can either promote or inhibit the processes of anticipatory grieving.

Pastors involved in the care of persons with AIDS will inevitably encounter aspects of anticipatory grieving. In some important ways, their interventions may catalyze and support these adaptive processes. Pastoral care not only helps a person deal effectively with the present, but it assists the individual to make peace with the past and prepare for the future. In the following case study, we shall consider some strategies of pastoral care which assist in this adaptive process.

Kent and Elaine Munley met when they were in graduate school. Kent had completed his first year of divinity studies and Elaine was in the second year of her graduate program in financial management. They dated and were married fourteen months later. After his ordination in the Episcopal Church, Kent was invited to become assistant rector in an affluent suburban community near New York City. Elaine found an excellent job and commuted daily from their home in Westchester County to her work in Manhattan. Kent and Elaine were well received by the church's congregation, and Kent was very happy in his first parish experience.

During the third year of Kent's ministry at Saint Matthew's, he developed a diarrheal infection, Cryptosporidiosis. At first he thought he had a simple intestinal virus. He used some over-the-counter medications, hoping to check the diarrhea. When the abdominal cramping persisted along with the symptoms of diarrhea, Kent sought the consultation of an internist. The physician was very concerned when he saw Kent. At the time of the examination, Kent was significantly dehydrated, had lost important body salts, and had lost almost ten pounds of body weight. In completing a detailed medical history, the AIDS-knowledgeable physician inquired of Kent's sexual history, and learned that Kent had been actively involved in anonymous homosexual experiences. Elaine had not been aware of these extramarital activities. The doctor, suspicious that Kent may have been exposed to the AIDS virus, examined his stool specifically for Cryptosporidium. The tiny protozoan parasite was detected. Kent's blood was simultaneously tested. Not only was he antibody positive for HIV, but his immunoglobulin level was well above average for a man of twenty-nine years of age. The physician told him that he had ARC.

Although there was insufficient evidence to make a definitive diagnosis of AIDS, it was not many months before his medical condition worsened. In the intervening months, Kent shared his story with Elaine, and with Rev. Byram Coolidge, the rector at Saint Matthew's. Kent was reluctant to involve his or Elaine's family who lived in other states. Kent initially believed that he would be able to manage his problems, and that with proper nutrition, exercise, and rest he would check the course of the disease. Elaine was shocked to learn of her husband's diagnosis, and hurt to discover his extramarital sexual history. Nonetheless, she was extraordinarily supportive of Kent, and encouraged him in his resolve to maintain his health. Rev. Coolidge was also understanding and helpful.

Five months after his initial presentation with Cryptosporidia, Kent was hospitalized. A bronchial biopsy examination verified a diagnosis of Pneumocystis carinii pneumonia. Kent had AIDS. At the time of his hospitalization he had shortness of breath and a hacking, dry cough, and was running a high fever. Upon admission his blood gases indicated that his blood was poorly oxygenated, and he required additional oxygen through a breathing tube.

During this crisis period, Kent began to deal with the realization that he might die from AIDS. It was with his colleague, Rev. Coolidge, that he began to voice his fears. Rev. Coolidge gently urged him to express whatever he wanted. Although Rev. Coolidge had been responsive from the start, Ken had not chosen to confide too much in his colleague. Now, with the incontrovertible indications that he had a full-blown case of AIDS, he was ready to use Coolidge's offers of help. It was a relief to Kent that Byram Coolidge was willing to become an active partner in this process and an important emotional support.

Kent admitted that he was reluctant to place additional burdens on his wife, since she already had more to bear than she was able to shoulder. How to tell their families about his diagnosis, what precisely to say, what their responses would be—all of these questions preoccupied Kent. He was worried about what would happen in the parish community and town when it would become known that the assistant rector of Saint Matthew's had AIDS. How would people react? Would Elaine be ostracized? Would she become infected? (Elaine has remained antibody negative for the AIDS virus in repeated tests.) These and other similar concerns dominated the early conversations between the two priests.

Coolidge was able to recognize some of the feelings associated with anticipatory grieving in Kent's behavior. Kent expressed his anger. The "Why me?" questions were voiced. He felt that he had tried to live a good life, despite his compulsive needs for anonymous sexual encounters. He directed his anger at God who he felt had abandoned him. Guilt was a natural counterpoint to his anger. "How could Elaine forgive him for his betrayal?" "How could God forgive him for putting himself in mortal danger by his irresponsible behavior?" "How could the bishop and Rev. Coolidge forgive him the scandal his illness would bring upon the Episcopal Church and the parish in which he served?" Kent vacillated between anger and blame, guilt and shame. In all of this he was physically and emotionally depressed. The pneumonia left him weak and unable to invest as much energy as he seemed to want in the conversations with Rev. Coolidge.

Byram Coolidge was a wise and caring older priest. He listened quietly and patiently. His facial expressions and gestures encouraged Kent to speak. When Kent finished, Rev. Coolidge would summarize many of the feelings Kent had verbalized. In a skillful way, Coolidge would begin to process these feelings, commenting upon them, responding to the effect he perceived. This required little of Kent, other than to listen. Rev. Coolidge always concluded a session with Kent by returning to prayer. He was comfortable vocalizing prayer, drawing upon many of the topics discussed in the conversation, or in previous meetings. What these experiences of prayer did for Kent was to help him maintain a sense of connectedness with God and with his friend.

Bereavement Needs of Unidentified Family Members

In common usage, we tend to think about bereavement in families in nuclear terms. Many of our examples throughout this book have focused on the ways in which spouses, parents, children and siblings have responded to another family member with AIDS. However, there have been many examples of non-family members who have had significant relationships with the sick or dying person. These relationships may include close friends, members of the clergy, a former spouse, a lover. However, not all significant persons have an opportunity to participate in the terminal care of a person with AIDS. Let us consider some of the problems associated with this reality.

Not all of the extrafamilial relationships we noted above receive the sanction and approval of the principal members of a family. A clear message may be communicated that these "non-family" members are not welcome to participate in the care of a person dying with AIDS. This is perhaps most commonly encountered with the gay lover of a person with AIDS.

Chris, the only son of Clara and Henry Burke, had been living away from home since his graduation from college in 1978. Although he was sure his parents suspected that he was gay, he perceived a clear but unstated message from them that they did not want to know. Henry Burke was a quiet man, and was characteristically non-verbal. Clara, on the other hand, was highly verbal. All important family discussions were mediated through Clara, and not through Henry. Anytime Chris got close to discussing the topic of his homosexuality with his mother she quickly changed the focus of the conversation. She always referred to Chris' lover, Ed, as his roommate. From every indication she gave, she did not like Ed, and was cool to him on every occasion that they met. When Chris confronted his mother about her attitudes toward Ed, she denied that she disliked him. But her behavior betrayed her disapproval.

When Chris became ill with AIDS-related symptoms in 1984, Clara became more directly involved in her son's life again. Although Ed wanted Chris to remain in their apartment, Chris was persuaded by his mother to come home. There was much tension in the relationship, but Chris did move home. Over the course of the next several months, Chris had an increasing number of infections and was hospitalized on three separate occasions. He was losing weight, had chronic diarrhea, suffered two major seizures, and contracted Pneumocystis pneumonia.

At first Clara allowed Ed to visit. As Chris' condition deteriorated, she was more resistant to Ed's involvement in Chris' care. She and Henry did not involve Ed in any decisions about their son's treatment. During his final weeks of life, Chris was mentally confused, and at times semi-conscious. Ed did not have adequate private time to say goodbye.

When Chris died, the Burkes did not invite Ed to participate in any specific way in planning the funeral. Ed was present at the funeral, but was not invited to sit with Clara and Henry, along with their other relatives and friends.

It was clear in this case that Clara and Henry could not cope with the acknowledgement that Chris and Ed had been lovers. Chris' prolonged dying from AIDS-related illnesses was extremely stressful on his parents, especially on his mother. She was not willing to accept the reality of her son's homosexuality, and was embarrassed by her son's illness. In her attempts to cope with these painful experiences, she excluded Ed from an appropriate place in the processes of anticipatory grieving. Ed was not permitted a role in Chris' terminal care or in the funeral rituals. As a result, Ed did not have an appropriate way in which to express or share his grief within the network of the Burke family. No one of Chris' other relatives expressed sympathy or condolences to Ed. In this sense, he was an unidentified person, excluded from societal support in his loss.

Days after Chris' funeral, Ed called and arranged an appointment with Father Timilty, the priest who had celebrated the funeral Mass. The priest's comforting words at the funeral helped Ed to risk initiating contact with him. As Ed, a non-Catholic, began to share with the priest some of the basic facts about his former relationship with Chris, he began to cry. The priest quickly assessed the situation and understood Ed's emotional needs. He encouraged Ed to express his feelings, and Father Timilty was accepting and responsive.

It was clear that Ed had bottled up much of his frustration and anger. He had lost his "best friend" in Chris, a confidant, the most significant person in his life. The priest did not underestimate the importance attached to Ed's descriptive comments. Ed had felt closed-out by the Burkes, distanced from Chris at a time when he knew Chris needed him the most. Ed felt guilty that he had abandoned Chris, that he had not stood up more forcefully to Mrs. Burke.

Over the next several weeks, Father Timilty had several good conversations with Ed. Through these conversations, Ed was able to reflect upon his life and relationship with Chris and process many of the feelings associated with his grief. Father Timilty legitimized Ed's grief by meeting with him and providing him a number of occasions in which he could work through his experiences of loss. Many times Father Timilty said to Ed: "I know that you were Chris' best friend, and that you loved each other very much." In retrospect, Ed said that the priest's acknowledgement of this relationship was the single statement that was most helpful to him in coping with the death of his lover. He also recalled that never once did Father Timilty speak judgmentally about the fact of their homosexual relationship, even though Ed assumed that the priest did not approve of that lifestyle. The issue simply never came up in their discussions.

Ed was very grateful that he had contacted Father Timilty, and that the priest was willing and capable of giving him support. He and the priest decided that it would not be productive to attempt reconciliation of the stressful relationship with the Burkes. Father Timilty was successful in assisting Ed to actively engage in the grief work which might otherwise have been blocked. Had not this important pastoral relationship been established, it is conceivable that Ed may have experienced extended depression stemming from guilt, anger, and other feelings associated with inhibited or unresolved grief work associated with the circumstances of Chris' death.

In cases like this, pastors should be alert to those important individuals who may not have sanctioned or recognized places in the family system, but whose relationship with the dying or deceased individual may put them at significant risk if they are excluded from appropriate support. Pastors who recognize and communicate with such individuals can be important resources to them. In the case mentioned above, Father Timilty concluded his formal meetings with Ed by conducting a brief memorial service, at which time Ed was given an appropriate forum to say his final goodbye to his friend. This single gesture helped Ed to reach closure on an important relationship in his life. Pastoral care was able to achieve what other interventions might not have been able to accomplish as effectively.

Pastoral Involvement with Bereaved Family Members

Throughout this book we have discussed various needs of individuals who provide care and support for a person with AIDS. We would now like to focus our attention on the specific bereavement needs of these same care-providers. A prolonged AIDS-related death taxes the physical and emotional reservoirs of family members, lovers, and friends who provide care. For a person dying with AIDS, this care brings the greatest degree of comfort and support. After the person has died, care-providers report that they derive considerable consolation in the knowledge that they did what they could to assist the dying person. However, bereaved family members and friends have special needs to which pastoral care can respond.

Bereavement can affect the physical and emotional health

of survivors. It is not uncommon that survivors experience a variety of bereavement-related complaints including anxiety and depression, personality and mood changes, and a range of psychophysiological symptoms. Some of these physical and emotional conditions become so serious that the bereaved person seeks the advice of physicians and mental health professionals. Clergy are often among those individuals to whom the bereaved turn for guidance and support.

The behavior of individual family members in response to the death of another member can be disruptive. An AIDS-related death may introduce changes in family structure to such an extent that families can be torn apart. The hospice philosophy of care includes bereavement follow-up as an integral component of its program of support. However, bereavement follow-up is not an ordinary part of routine medical care. Few physicians and nurses see their responsibilities extending to family members beyond the death of a patient. In the AIDS pandemic, the limited resources of hospital and other professional staff are being stretched to their full limits. This situation often leaves families without the kind of professional assistance they frequently need as they attempt to resume their lives after the death of a loved one.

The Sullivan family exemplifies the problem we have been exploring. Kathleen and Jerome Sullivan had four children: three daughters and one son. Terry Sullivan, their only son, had graduated from law school and was practicing in a large urban center in the northeastern United States. When Terry was diagnosed with AIDS in the summer of 1985, he chose to become public about his illness. Although he had been hospitalized several times during the last year of his life, Terry spoke at many seminars on the disease, calling for more public awareness and compassion for persons with AIDS. He produced a videotape which he hoped would be useful in AIDS-related educational efforts. As it turned out, Terry died several days after the video was completed.

Terry's sisters were accepting and supportive of their brother, encouraging him in his decision to make his disease an issue of public education. His sisters themselves became active in AIDS education activities. Mr. and Mrs. Sullivan did not respond favorably. They disapproved of the public attention Terry's illness brought to the family. They were embarrassed by Terry's disclosure. His parents did not participate in any of Terry's activities prior to his death, and were critical of the ways in which their daughters were championing Terry's activist approach to AIDS. His parents were involved minimally in his illness, preferring to maintain a distance.

After Terry's death, the parents were angered when their daughters elected to continue the work that Terry had begun in AIDS education. Terry's sisters utilized their brother's videotape as they spoke at numerous AIDS awareness seminars organized by various civic and church groups. In reaction the parents put their home on the market, sold many of their family possessions, and moved to an undisclosed location. Effectively, they cut themselves off from their family.

Throughout this family crisis, the Sullivans never sought support from their pastor. They were reluctant to involve the Church in their son's illness because he had abandoned the practice of Roman Catholicism and considered himself to be a Quaker. For themselves, the parents were embarrassed to talk about their own feelings and reactions with a priest. As a result, they were isolated in their bereavement. Not only did their son die of AIDS, but they lost all important relationships with their other children. Terry's death was the occasion for a major family split.

The Sullivans' pastor did not intervene in the family's crisis. It is likely that had he taken some initiative, the chasm of alienation and separation might not have become as pronounced. Pastoral care could have helped the parents work with the stigma and guilt they felt as a result of Terry's public identification as a person with AIDS. Separated from the important sources of support of family and Church, Kathleen and Jerome Sullivan themselves became victims of AIDS. For them, their grief and bereavement encompassed not only the death of a son, but the loss of their home, family, and friends. This is a senseless tragedy which might have been avoided with appropriate interventions.

In this case, we have introduced once again the issue of stigma. We explored the issue of stigma earlier in the discussion of the psychosocial needs of persons with AIDS. Stigma always plays some part in a person's reaction to bereavement. Societies respond to death and bereavement in different ways. For many of us, it is disquieting to be in the presence of someone who has recently experienced the death of a loved one. We do not know what to say. We are reluctant to raise the topic of the death for fear that it might be painful for the bereaved.

The circumstances of the loved one's death can either lessen or intensify the ways in which others respond. If the death was the result of AIDS, this might create other barriers for surviving family members. Families of persons who have died of AIDS experience this stigma. Not only are they the parents, widows, siblings, or lovers of a person who has died, but they are the ones who survive a person who died of AIDS. The fact of an AIDS-related death contributes to the alienation and isolation experienced by the bereaved. If it is common for people to avoid the recently bereaved, then it should not be surprising that avoidance of survivors of persons who died of AIDS will be more pronounced.

Some families have talked about feeling contaminated, as if others think they could catch the disease by simple association. Siblings report that they sense being avoided or ostracized in many business and social environments if the cause of a relative's death from AIDS is known. The stigma of AIDS carries beyond the grave for surviving family members.

Just as widows have turned to other widows for support (Widow-to-Widow), and bereaved parents have looked for assistance from other parents who have lost children (Compassionate Friends), family members of persons with AIDS have found it necessary to group together with other families in order to cope with their grief. In these self-help groups of persons with similar experiences, bereaved individuals do not feel stigmatized. They find understanding, acceptance, guidance, and support. Groups such as Mothers of AIDS Patients (MAP), the National Association of People with AIDS (NAPWA), and the Parents and Friends of Lesbians and Gays (PFLAG) have been responsive to the particular needs of families who have lost a member to AIDS.

Pastoral care should never consciously contribute to the

stigma associated with survivors of an AIDS death. Pastors can be helpful liaisons in bridging the distance that separates a bereaved family from others within the community.

Mending the Loss

At the outset of this chapter, we defined grief as a normal response and reaction to loss. The loss of a loved one engages the processes of grieving. However, another component of loss involves dealing with the deprivation occasioned by the loss. Relationships with certain people provide important physical and psychological supports to individuals. For example, one person may be a confidant, a trusted critic, a prudent counselor, and a lover. If that individual dies, the survivor is deprived of these important psychological supports. The normal response to deprivation is loneliness.

One of the difficulties in dealing with deprivation is that people are not always articulate in defining what specific supports were surrendered in the death of a loved one. It is not uncommon to find bereaved persons laconic when it comes to naming the specific ways in which the death of a loved one has deprived the survivor of important physical and emotional supports. Colin Murray Parkes, a psychiatric pioneer in bereavement research, has often compared deprivation in situations of loss to having food and water withheld. Just as these latter supplies are essential to physical functioning, many of the emotional supplies provided in human relationships are essential to psychological functioning.

In his diary of the progress of his own grieving, *A Grief Observed* (1961), C.S. Lewis provides a clear example of what he felt deprived in the death of his wife.

> For a good wife contains so many persons in herself. What was H. not to me? She was my daughter and my mother, my pupil and my teacher, my subject and my sovereign; and always, holding all these in solution, my trusty comrade, friend, shipmate, fellow-soldier. My mistress; but at the same time all that any man friend (and I have good

ones) has ever been to me. Perhaps more. If we had never fallen in love we should have none the less been always together, and created a scandal. . . . (p. 39)

Did you ever know, dear, how much you took away with you when you left? You have stripped me even of my past, even of the things we never shared. I was wrong to say the stump was recovering from the pain of amputation. I was deceived because it has so many ways to hurt me that I discover them only one by one. (p. 48)

For C.S. Lewis, the notebooks in which he recorded his personal account of grieving became a vehicle for processing his loss. He was able to articulate the specific deprivations he felt as a result of his wife's death. One of the tasks of grief work is to find alternative sources for the lost supports. The loneliness, frustration, insecurity, and other emotions commonly associated with bereavement can be expected to continue as long as the survivor remains deprived.

Pastoral intervention with any bereaved individual needs to address the sources of deprivation as well as attend to other secondary losses, role changes, and stigma associated with the death of a loved one. In working with the survivors of persons who have died of AIDS, there are some specific tasks which pastoral care may be in the best position to address.

If a pastor has been effective in ministering to a person with AIDS who has died, then it is reasonable that he or she may be invited to extend ministerial support to bereaved survivors. It is not unusual that bereaved persons will turn for leadership and support to clergy who shared with them in the death of a loved one.

Rev. Jennifer Schultz, an Episcopal priest, was an integral part of the terminal illness of Jason Ross. She was chaplain at the hospital in which Jason died of respiratory failure associated with a primary diagnosis of AIDS. For the last few days of his life, Jason was placed on a respirator. At his own request and with the support of his lover, Michael, his parents, and other members of his immediate family, the medical staff disconnected the respirator and Jason died within minutes. Rev. Schultz was present with the family when Jason died.

Michael felt very close to the priest and sought her support not only during the period of the funeral, but in the weeks and months after Jason's death. We would like to focus on the pastor's short-term work with Michael, even though she was likewise helpful to other members of Jason's family who turned to her for guidance during the period of their bereavement.

One of the most important activities that Rev. Schultz encouraged Michael to undertake was to verbalize his feelings about Jason. In addition to giving words to his pain, sorrow, and loss, Michael also spoke at considerable length about his guilt. He felt guilty because he felt he had not been as supportive to Jason in his long struggle with AIDS as he could have been. He felt guilty that Jason was dead, and he, Michael, was still alive. During their early conversations, Rev. Schultz encouraged Michael and listened to many variations of the refrain: "If only I had . . ."

Rev. Schultz facilitated Michael's necessary review of the fourteen-year relationship that he and Jason had maintained. Meeting during their final year in college, Michael and Jason had been lovers for the major years of their young adult lives. At thirty-five years of age, Michael felt he had invested much in his relationship with Jason, and was angry that his friend had died. Reverend Schultz in her low-keyed way was able to help Michael to identify the most important deprivations associated with the loss of his lover. She was able to bolster Jason's self-esteem by her understanding and appreciation of the genuine love and commitment that had characterized the relationship between the two men. As Michael reviewed his relationship with Jason, Rev. Schultz was attentive and responsive. She actively reinforced the positive dimensions of his relationship with Jason, particularly when Michael began to dwell on how he had failed Jason. Her work with Michael helped him to achieve a balance between the positive and negative aspects of his long-term relationship with his deceased lover.

Michael found in Rev. Schultz a trusted confidante. He was able to share with her his emotional reactions to Jason's death. He told her about his hallucinations, believing that he heard Jason's voice or felt him in his bed. He told her that he was worried about his own weight loss, due to the fact that he was not eating properly. She was able to help him to understand that these were among normal psychophysiological reactions that a bereaved person experiences. He seemed to feel reassured simply because she told him it was normal.

During Jason's long illness, Michael's day-to-day routine was significantly altered. He found it difficult attempting to resume a normal schedule. Taking care of Jason had consumed a major part of his time, disrupting both his work and his recreation rhythm. He found it difficult to reintegrate himself into life without Jason. At times Michael felt bitter that he was now alone, did not feel attractive, and was despondent. Rev. Schultz encouraged him to assume greater responsibility for his reintegration into the mainstream of life.

As a hospital chaplain, Rev. Schultz provided a much needed service to Michael Reeves. In the six visits she had with Michael after Jason's death she was able to help him work with a number of important and practical issues pertaining to his grief work. As the homosexual lover of a person who died of AIDS, Michael was in a vulnerable position, with few potential sources of effective help available to him. As a chaplain who had been supportive to Jason and his family during his final hospitalization, Rev. Schultz was in an optimal position to support the family in the important work of their grieving. That Michael sought and utilized well her assistance is evident from the few details of this case summary. Clergy should not be reluctant to offer assistance to bereaved family members. Should their interventions not be effective, they can be instrumental in seeking other medical and/or psychiatric support for the bereaved.

Putting to Use Old Griefs

In one of Elizabeth Barrett Browning's *Sonnets to the Portuguese,* she writes of her love for Robert, saying, "I love thee with all the passion put to use in my old griefs." Certainly, the most significant human crisis that most of us face in life is the death of a loved one. For many, it is a radical event, necessitating changes in many aspects of living. In this book we have described many lives changed and lost by AIDS. We have shared the experiences of spouses and children, parents and siblings, lovers and friends whose lives have been altered by the HIV antibody status or the confirmation of AIDS in a loved one.

When a person dies of an AIDS-related disease, the bereaved survivor's life can move in one of two directions. It can constrict or expand, regress or move on. The bereaved individual can remain isolated in despair or can find new hope, new meaning, and purpose in the loss. In the poet's words, the bereaved can harness the experience of loss and put to use his or her old griefs.

We have seen some remarkable examples of this harnessing of grief in the survivors of persons who have died of AIDS. People like Barbara Peabody (*A Screaming Room*), BettyClare Moffatt (*When Someone You Love Has AIDS: A Book of Hope for Family and Friends*), and Carol Lynn Pearson (*Good-Bye, I Love You*) represent a growing group of individuals who have put to use their grief. Some of these survivors have been instrumental in organizing groups to support other parents and loved ones as they struggle to care for a person living and dying with AIDS. Others are focusing their grief on advocacy issues for other persons with AIDS. Like the Sullivan sisters who took up their deceased brother's mission, despite the cost it had in terms of relationship with their parents, bereaved individuals are putting their grief to work in AIDS educational efforts in the wider social community.

Clergy who minister to individuals who are dying of AIDS and to their bereaved survivors experience grief as well. Such grief, however, contributes to our becoming more human. It makes us more understanding, accepting, and compassionate. We cannot enter the lives of persons who are dying of AIDS and remain unaffected by that experience. Being admitted into the hopes and sorrows of a person dying of AIDS and his or her family teaches the minister much about human love and commitment. Sharing the grief of survivors makes the minister more sensitive, more responsive, more loving. Grief has a positive side for clergy who experience it as a result of their own investment in the lives of families coping with an AIDS-related death.

In a genuine sense, this book grows out of the grief I have personally experienced in ministry to individuals living with the ever-present reality that they are dying of AIDS and those loved ones who survive them. Grief has motivated me to reinvest my own energies and experiences, first released in sorrow, but rechannelled into work with other care-providers who share this important ministry.

The Ministry of Listening

There is an old saying that could easily become a motto for pastoral care of the bereaved: "When in doubt, listen." Too many pastors think that they need to verbally respond to everything a bereaved person feels or says. Pastoral care with the bereaved has a number of specific goals, many of which we have been discussing. A principal goal is helping the survivor with the difficult agenda of accepting the loss. As a person gradually comes to this acceptance, he or she will frequently verbalize many things. Much of what is said by a bereaved person does not require verbal response. In fact, if a pastor gets too involved in discussion, he or she may distract the bereaved from important agendas.

Throughout our discussion of grief and bereavement, we have placed significant emphasis on the expression of feeling. By our privileged positions in the lives of dying persons and their families, people come to trust that they can dare to express to us feelings that they might otherwise withhold from others. When people are hurting, as most bereaved acknowledge they do, a pastor is an important resource in encouraging and absorbing these feelings. Once again, the role of the pastor is more often receiver than transmitter.

A pastor's receptivity, understanding, and encouragement can help the bereaved person to cry and to express the range of ambivalent feelings associated with the illness and death of the loved one. As a bereaved person expresses his or her feelings some pastors become defensive, judgmental, and rejecting. These inappropriate and negative responses become additional burdens for a bereaved person. Because the individual is emotionally vulnerable, perceived attack and rejection by a pastor is experienced as a significant wound. In some cases, perceived rejection by a pastor may inhibit a bereaved individual's normal processes of grieving.

If the environment is perceived as receptive and understanding, a bereaved individual will gradually talk about the loss. In some of the pastoral cases we have presented, we have seen how freely some individuals will talk about intimate details of a lost relationship. It is not unusual that conversation tends to be very self-centered. The bereaved person will often be preoccupied with thoughts about his or her own life without the deceased loved one. Pastoral care of the bereaved is frequently a bridge to the future. A bereaved person needs to consider how he or she will resume living after the death of the loved one. For all of this, a bereaved person needs a sensitive ear.

For some individuals experiencing loss, the person of the pastor is seen as the stillpoint in a topsy-turvy world. The pastor represents stability in an environment of many changes. Many individuals look to pastors for temporary anchorage. If the pastor has been with the family during the extended crisis from diagnosis to ultimate death, he or she is a logical person to see the family through its period of acute grief and adjustment. A pastor can help a family to be patient with its adjustments and judicious in making the changes that are part of accepting the loss of a loved one.

The Role of Pastoral Ministry
in Bereavement Outreach

Managing grief takes time, but it is an active process. Pastors can be helpful in encouraging bereaved persons to network with others in similar situations. Local AIDS task forces and AIDS Action Committees in many cities and towns are developing resources to assist the survivors of persons who have died of AIDS. Resolving one's loss is often linked to resuming the normal activities of one's life. As mentioned earlier, a support group can often be instrumental in helping a person to reengage with normal living.

The philosophy of living one day at a time is made more manageable when a person perceives that he or she has support. In caring for a person with AIDS, one appropriates this philosophy of life. Each day contains its own specific agenda. This same reality is descriptive of dealing with grief. Persons who have completed the major work of grieving can be helpful to others who are just beginning.

Churches can be instrumental in bringing people together. There are many resources that bereaved people may not know that they have. Mothers of young people who have died of AIDS can be comforting and supportive of other parents in similar circumstances. Other persons who have lost a loved one to AIDS can be helpful to the friends and lovers recently bereaved. Nothing is more therapeutic than to be able to care about another person. It seems to bring meaning to one's own personal sorrow, one's own sense of loss. Reaching out to other persons, embracing them in their experiences of grief, helps the helper to move beyond his or her own personal loss.

If religion has had some place in the life of the deceased and his or her family, then the churches can be important resources in outreach after the person has died. The religious services organized by churches to support persons with AIDS and their care-providers, and the rituals that have been celebrated to commemorate those who have died of AIDS, have been helpful. In managing grief, religious faith can be a powerful ally. Through spiritual ministries, the churches can reach out to the community of the bereaved in unique and effective ways. Ironically, this resource may be underutilized, but its potential value to bereaved persons should never be underestimated.

For example, in Chicago, men and women professionals from different faith traditions, who are trained to offer pastoral care to their sisters and brothers who are affected directly and indirectly by AIDS, have formed the AIDS Pastoral Care Network. This interfaith group makes faith and spirituality effective resources in this time of crisis. This outreach program ministers to persons with AIDS and ARC and their loved ones by providing pastoral services, counseling, and liturgical services as appropriate. In its mission statement, the AIDS Pastoral Care Network notes that its ministry to affected communities, care-givers, and society "stems from our commitment to educate them about the pastoral, spiritual, and religious implications of AIDS and to provide direct pastoral services to them when these are needed."

The philosophy of the AIDS Pastoral Care Network maintains that authentic pastoral care proceeds from a wholeness that addresses political and religious issues, avoidable and un-avoidable suffering, social justice, and pastoral care. The group's mission statement further operationalizes this principle of pastoral care. "As pastoral ministers we are committed to work for social justice because we are aware that prejudice, discrimination, and alienation have increased in unconscionable ways the already heavy burden of suffering of people affected by AIDS." Pastoral volunteers see their roles as embracing both direct service and advocacy. In this latter role, the AIDS Pastoral Care Network plays an assertive role in opposing actions of those leaders or institutions which adversely affect the people with whom and for whom they minister.

Among the services provided by volunteers within this network is support to all affected persons in love and faith. The spiritual ministries of prayer and liturgical gatherings not only are sources of healing and reconciliation for persons directly affected by the disease, but they can be very beneficial to bereaved loved ones. Fr. Carl Meirose, S.J., Executive Director of the AIDS Pastoral Care Network, recognizes that among the group's priorities, spirituality is an important resource to persons with AIDS and their loved ones.

This model interfaith collaborative ministry, founded in 1985, is but one example of the Church taking a proactive role in the AIDS crisis. It has drawn together sensitive pastoral care volunteers, clerics and lay, to bring the churches' healing ministries to persons with AIDS and ARC, their families, lovers, and friends. As a comprehensive ministry, the follow-up work with the bereaved is an important component of its ministry.

In the Book of Psalms we read: "I lift up my eyes to the mountains: where is help to come from? Help comes to me from Yahweh, who made heaven and earth" (Ps 121:1–2). To the audible and silent cries of those who mourn a loved one who has died from this devastating group of diseases called AIDS, where is help to come from? Certainly, it must come from those whose public profession is identified with the compassionate face of God. The psalmist continues: "Yahweh guards you, shades you; with Yahweh at your right hand sun cannot strike you down by day, nor moon at night. Yahweh guards you from harm, he guards your lives, he guards you leaving, coming back, now and for always" (Ps 21:5–8). Pastoral care is a privileged expression of God's love and protection for those who mourn. Blessed are they who mourn, for they shall be comforted. Blessed, too, are the comforters—the pastors who love them, listen to them, accept them, attempt to understand their feelings until quietness, new hope, and new life return.